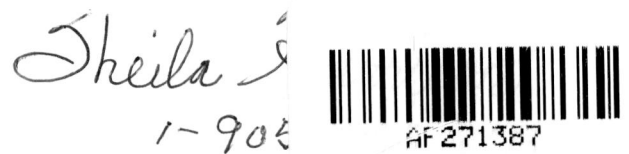
THE EARTH'S GIFT TO MEDICINE

Minerals in Health and Disease

A Source Book for Doctors and Patients
Foreword by Dr. Abram Hoffer

Klaus-Georg Wenzel
Raymond J. Pataracchia

Note: Although this book is intended for professionals and the general public, it is not to be used as a replacement for medical advice.

Medicine is constantly evolving through research and experience. It is not unusual, even in other fields, that new knowledge includes contradictory findings. Sometimes, these contradictions lead to new findings. Even though our present knowledge may be complemented or discharged in the future, it is important to pause and gain an overview of what has currently been found.

This book makes use of information from different sources and countries. In some cases, references are made to theoretical items which have not been fully proven, or which have only been reported by individual sources. Such information is included when it has been judged by the authors to be of theoretical or practical importance.

For correspondence please contact:

Dr. med. Klaus-Georg Wenzel
Diezer Strasse 14
Germany, 65549 Limburg
Email: Dr.Wenzel@Dr-Wenzel.com

Dr. Raymond J Pataracchia B.Sc., N.D.
441-20 Eglinton Ave. E.
Toronto, Ontario, Canada, M4P 1A9
Tel: 416-944-8824
E-mail: info@nmrc.ca
Website: www.nmrc.ca

TABLE OF CONTENTS

Minerals listed in bold are more commonly used in clinical practice.
Latin names appear in parentheses.

Section 2

FOREWORD BY ABRAM HOFFER

The vast importance of trace elements in maintaining health in all living tissue was recognized several hundred years ago when the role of iron was understood. Over the past 100 years, the roles of all the trace elements, their properties and side effects, how much must be used, and the dangers of taking too much have been discovered. Adding iodide to ordinary table salts prevents epidemics of goiter caused by soils that are terribly deficient. Agriculturists, botanists and anyone who loves to grow flowers knows about the importance of these trace elements to their plants. Plants are happy if provided with a place in which to grow, with water, sunlight and minerals, which they cannot make. They can make everything else that they need. Animals from the lowest protozoa to humans are equally dependent on minerals, which must be provided. We cannot make minerals nor can we make a small number of organic substances called vitamins. By freeing ourselves of the need to make everything, by learning that we can eat plants that have what we need (food), we have gained mobility and speech but we have become dependent on plant forms for the minerals, vitamins and essential fatty acids. We know how important minerals are, especially calcium related to osteoporosis, iron for our hemoglobin, and iodine for our thyroid glands, but we still have not realized the vast importance of other trace minerals such as selenium in dealing with viral infections, and zinc and copper in dealing with some psychoses. This very good book summarizes the properties of 39 minerals, the good as well as the bad.

Over the past 30 years I have reviewed several hundred books in this new field of nutritional medicine. Of these, two dealing with minerals stand out: the first by Carl Pfeiffer, called *Mental and Elemental Nutrients* published in 1975, and this one. This book is well organized and reads well. For each mineral the left hand page lists the normal daily requirements, functions, therapeutic applications, negative biological effects and sources. And on the right hand page we find discussions of how each mineral works, why it is needed and so on. As an example, selenium. The review of selenium by the authors is comprehensive. I selected selenium because its importance in dealing with viral epidemics such as HIV has not yet been recognized.

These two authors tell us that selenium was discovered in 1817 and was first used for treating inoperable tumors in the 1930's and 1940's with success. In 1957, it was proven to be essential. Its usefulness is becoming increasingly recognized. In Finland, selenium has been added to grain since

1984. 200 µg is about the daily requirement. I use up to 1000 µg as part of the treatment for cancer. Deficiency arises on water-washed soils, which have benefited the oceans by transferring selenium from the land to the sea. Its deficiency is implicated in a number of conditions, which I think ought simply to be called selenium deficiency diseases. In China, for example, its absence causes Keshan disease. Selenium is needed for the immune system; it has antioxidant properties; and more. It is a component of glutathione peroxidase, an essential enzyme in the body. It is necessary for production of thyroid hormone. Toxicity in small doses has been exaggerated in the past but it is now recognized that there is no toxicity in the recommended dose range.

I do recommend that every person dealing with health have this book in his or her library and by his or her side. Physicians who pay attention to the properties of these minerals and use them in their practices will be surprised and pleased at how much better their patients will be.

Dr. Abram Hoffer, M.D., Ph.D.

ACKNOWLEDGEMENTS

It takes a long time and a lot of friends to write a book. I want to thank Claudia Rank, a naturopathic medical student in Toronto, for translating this book from its original German; David Sealey, B.Sc., (Ph.D. Candidate) in Toronto, for his excellent editing work on the English translation; and Keith Boa, from Toronto, for the graphic design and general production of the final text.

I also want to thank my co-author Raymond J. Pataracchia N.D. for having given me the idea to translate and adapt the German original for North American readers. We first met at a conference of the International Association for Orthomolecular Medicine (ISOM) in Toronto at which I presented a lecture on orthomolecular medicine in psychiatry. Subsequently, Dr. Pataracchia visited me at my clinic in Germany as a part of his medical training.

Over the past year, Robert Sealey gave excellent support in coordinating all our joint efforts for this project and also found a Canadian publisher, Kos Publishing Inc.

My daughter Nicole Wenzel – who just finished her university education and practices veterinary medicine, often gave me important and helpful hints from her field: it is a most interesting fact that in veterinary medicine trace elements (minerals, vitamins and other essential nutrients) are considered of vital importance and represent an integral part of the daily practice of animal doctors. Veterinarians know of the vital importance of these essential nutrients in the treatment of many diseases and of their significance in all metabolic processes. I would like this awareness to become part of all of medicine.

Very special thanks are for my wife Ursula who often supported me and had a lot of understanding when I was working on the book for so many hours – thank you, I love you.

I also thank my patients who helped me to develop a better understanding of disease and health. Of course, there are many more friends and colleagues whose knowledge and inspirations have always been and still are important to me in my never-ending desire to improve my skills in helping my patients.

Chinese wisdom informs us that one never reaches a goal in life, but the pursuit of the goal, the Tao is the goal. There will never be an end to learning.

Klaus Wenzel, March 2005

PUBLISHER'S PREFACE*

Every publisher loves having a manuscript dropped on them that is fabulous and totally unexpected. This book is both. Its English translation from the German original was sent to me by my friend Robert Sealey with whom I share a deep appreciation for clinical nutrition and the work of Dr. Abram Hoffer who together with Linus Pauling initiated this branch of medicine. The authors employ the principles of lab-based nutritional medicine in their practices, and so I knew at once that this book would be a gold mine for Kos readers – indeed, the appropriate metaphor for a book on minerals. The gold I refer to is the information this book contains for all those seeking health which, only medicine that works in harmony with nature, can deliver. Dr. Klaus-Georg Wenzel is a psychiatrist and neurologist practicing in Germany, and Dr. Pataracchia is a Canadian naturopathic doctor. They produced a most informative book on the importance of minerals for the prevention and treatment of disease which will delight patients and medical practitioners alike. Here you will learn how minerals work, which minerals make your life and health possible, and which minerals are toxic and must be removed and avoided.

Some years back I interviewed Dr. Abram Hoffer and he made a comment that had a profound impression on me: "Doctors are not trained as scientists. They are not trained in chemistry. They are not trained to understand health and disease as biochemical processes." To my delight, I learned that Dr. Wenzel had a hard time deciding whether to become a doctor or a chemist, having tinkered in his own personal laboratory since high school. This book shows how scientific thinking is helpful when seeking to understand dynamic interactions and biochemical individuality versus simplistic explanations for complex problems.

As a medical student Dr. Wenzel visited the US where he first came into contact with research into and on the application of trace minerals in clinical practice. He also learned about the work of Dr. Abram Hoffer and Linus Pauling who spearheaded this approach to health and disease. He became a member of the International Society for Orthomolecular Medicine and has since then, attended almost every ISOM annual conference. This year, at the 34th annual conference (May 12-15, 2005) in Ottawa, Kos Publishing will also launch Dr. Abram Hoffer's autobiography (visit the Kos website at www. kospublishing.com).

The second author of this book, Dr. Raymond Pataracchia, following his training in neuroscience became a naturopathic doctor; naturopathy has for centuries focused on therapies that utilize trace minerals and nutritional therapies to address chronic and acute pathology.

I am personally especially interested in disseminating the information about the healing properties of minerals because minerals are really wonderful in the sense that they are such simple inorganic structures which yet have such vast biological implications. Consider that they are indeed the gift of the earth to organic life. Minerals are inorganic matter – the very stuff of the earth - yet, they become the most powerful catalysts for life itself when they act within an organism.

Billions of years ago, when the universe gave birth to unknown millions of galaxies, our planet eventually also appeared. The same star dust that became Earth, also created all life and maintains it every second of the day. Nobel laureate Christian de Duve writes, "All organic matter can be summarized by the formula CHNOPS, which stands for carbon, hydrogen, nitrogen, oxygen, phosphorus, and sulfur." If life was a symphony orchestra in which all instruments are equally important to the musical event - the players being vitamins, enzymes, proteins, hormones, and so on, the minerals would assume the role of the first violinist who presents the correct key-note to enable the conductor to begin. Thus, everything living and non-living is at every moment literally part of the earth as well as itself.

Andre Voisin, a French agricultural biochemist, who outlined the "principles of protective medicine, the great medical science of the future", observed in the 1950's, in his magisterial book *Soil, Grass and Cancer:* "We should frequently meditate on the words of Ash Wednesday: Man, remember that you are dust and that you will return to dust. This great scientific truth should be engraved above the entrance of every faculty of medicine ... [because] our cells are made up of mineral elements ... the animal is a product of the soil, the biochemical photograph of the environment in which it lives, particularly of the soil which manufactured the nutrients for it." Minerals are the catalysts of all biological activity where the boundary between organic and inorganic vanishes.

In 1920 - before the devil's brew of synthetic fertilizers, pesticides, herbicides, industrial chemicals, and acid rain - 50 bushels of grain contained the protein that by 1968 would be found in 100 bushels of grain; the vitamins found in 50 bushels then, by 1968 required 250 bushels; those 50 bushels of grain in 1920 were chock-full of essential minerals, but by 1968 it required 500 bushels for people to obtain the same mineral content. In March 2001, the US Department of Agriculture food tables showed that the amount of calcium (the king of minerals) in broccoli dropped by 50% from 1975 and the amount of iron in watercress dropped by 88%. The vitamin C content in sweet peppers dropped from an average of 128 mg to 89 mg; the potassium content in all foods dropped from 400 mg to 170 mg; and the magnesium level (the queen of minerals) dropped from 57% to 9%. By the way, if your serum level of magnesium drops on any day by a mere 10%, you may have a heart attack – the less dramatic, every-day low levels merely set us up for one. Conventionally grown potatoes and apples now have very little or no vitamin C or potassium at all (*Nature*, April 19, 2001).

The *American Journal of Clinical Nutrition* warned in 1999 (L. Chasen-Taber, 70:509-16) that the currently low levels of selenium predispose us to cancer. On July 3 the *Toronto Star's* front-page headline read "Cancer crisis looming in GTA" and reported a 46% predicted increase over the next ten years. It is well-known that continual exposure to environmental carcinogens and nutritionally dead food inhibits cell repair and, lowers our body's defense systems. This has been cited as a primary causative factor in cancer (*New England Journal of Medicine* July 13, 2000).

The US National Academy of Sciences issued an alert in 2004 stating that we have to double our intake of vegetables just to approximate the RDAs – which are themselves not in accord with the current body of scientific knowledge, being based on what a healthy male around age 18 may require. A world survey undertaken by The World Resources Institute in Washington DC, published March 2000, entitled *Underfed and Overfed*, discussed the "global epidemic of malnutrition", showing that the poor do not receive the required nutrients, because they lack the calories or food diversity, while the affluent are increasingly obese but are equally deprived of the same nutrients due to plentiful, instantly available, and perfect-looking food which is mostly nutritionally dead.

These minerals, which are the guardians of life, are primarily depleted by synthetic fertilizers, pesticides, herbicides, acid rain, and agricultural methods that have ceased to be in dialogue with the earth because of their exclusive focus on quantity, efficiency, and profit. One effect of ignoring the earth as the matrix of life is the depletion of those minerals which animals and people need in order to make catalase – the enzyme needed to prevent incorrect cell duplication, or cancer. Recently, University of British Columbia's medical geographer, Harold Foster discussed how, for example, Senegal with its naturally selenium-rich soils has almost no AIDS at all, even though the culture tolerates promiscuity, while certain parts of China are naturally selenium depleted and AIDS is heavily prevalent. In industrialized countries, the AIDS rate is highest where foods are lowest in selenium due to food processing and selenium-depleting agricultural methods. In 2004, the Ontario College of Family Physicians published their report on the health effects of pesticides, insisting they be stopped and urging people to eat organic food to ensure that the basic needs for minerals and other essential nutrients are met.

The Earth will never forsake us. You are invited to learn and apply this knowledge in your lives and professional work. Enjoy.

By Helke Ferrie

Sources:

C. Dean, MD, ND, *Death By Modern Medicine,* Matrix Verite, 2005

C. DeDuve, *Vital Dust: Life as A Cosmic Imperative,* Basic Books, 1995

H. Ferrie, *Dispatches from the War Zone of Environmental Health,* Kos, 2004

H. Foster, *What Really Causes AIDS,* Trafford, 2001

J. Krop, MD, *Healing The Planet One Patient At A Time,* 2nd edition, Kos, 2003

W. A. Price, *Nutrition and Physical Degeneration,* 50th anniversary edition, Keats, 1989

World Resources Institute Monograph 150: *Underfed and Overfed; The Global Epidemic of Malnutrition,* March 2000

A. Voisin, *Soil Grass and Cancer,* Crosby Lockwood Ltd., 1959 (out of print, for facsimile copies call Bio-Ag 519-656-2460)

* Parts of this preface are taken from an article I wrote for Vitality Magazine in October 2004

INTRODUCTION

Scientific and medical researchers have made many fascinating discoveries about trace elements. Many of these elements are essential to life, but some are harmful. Trace minerals discoveries have been recognized at an international level in academic medicine, yet some medical institutions often get so caught up with specific research projects that they miss the significance of the trace element field. Trace elements and minerals should not be trivialized as unimportant or overrated as miracle cures.

The bulk of knowledge on trace minerals is mainly derived from the US and Canada where their clinical application is more common. This is partly due to the fact that everyday medicine and research have more liberty in North America than in Europe where there are many bureaucratic and economic restrictions. When a treatment is proven effective, it is often put to use to help patients and to meet a market niche. Because the American diet is often inadequate and greatly influenced by fast food, many clinical problems present in the population as a result of trace mineral imbalances. Accordingly, a wide array of supplements and trace minerals are available in supermarkets and nutrition stores. However, poor labeling and advertising standards leave consumers and health professionals without adequate knowledge of product constituents and safety. Further, supplement manufacturers and distributors often use excessive marketing techniques. Consumers and physicians need to understand the appropriate uses for trace minerals. This book is designed to serve this purpose.

This book outlines those minerals most commonly used in clinical practice and those minerals that, in given situations, are considered detrimental to our health and well-being. Minerals commonly used in clinical practice include calcium, chromium, copper, iron, iodine, lithium, magnesium, manganese, molybdenum, potassium, selenium, sodium, and zinc. Minerals that can be detrimental to our health and well-being are toxic even in small doses - especially arsenic, cadmium, beryllium, mercury, lead, platinum, tin and thallium.

At the beginning of the last century, only minerals such as calcium that were present in large amounts in the human body could be measured. Many other chemical elements found in nature are present in such small amounts that they were not measurable. It was unknown whether they were present in the body by chance or whether they were essential for life. Naturally, not every element present in the body is required for us to live.

Some of the first elements recognized as 'essential to life'			
Iron	17-18th Century	Copper	1928
Magnesium	1931	Zinc	1934
Iodine	1950	Molybdenum	1953
Selenium	1957	Chromium	1959

Besides these "classic" essential trace elements, several others have been identified within the last 20-30 years as being required by humans in trace amounts (e.g. silicon). However, vanadium has not yet been universally confirmed as essential even though 20-40 mg is present in an adult body.

In general, minerals are found in an adult body in amounts exceeding 1 g, whereas anything present in a lesser amount is classified a trace element. For example, the 4 g of iron and the 2-3 g of zinc found in adults are considered minerals whereas iodine and the relatively unknown essential elements selenium and molybdenum, with 10-30 µg each, are examples of trace elements. Throughout medical history, the terms minerals and trace elements arose within a very limited detection system. Today, their distinction is somewhat arbitrary. Due to the arbitrary assignment and unclear distinction between minerals and trace elements, the term 'trace mineral' or 'trace element' seems appropriate. These terms bring forward the collective and synergistic nature of the periodic table of elements. This trace element concept is therefore clinically useful. In this book, to avoid confusion, the terms mineral, element, trace mineral, and trace element have been used interchangeably.

Selenium is an example of a trace element that is necessary for humans and animals, but not necessary for plants. This explains why plants can thrive in selenium-deficient soils (in China for example), whereas humans and animals can die under these conditions. On the other hand, harmful substances such as lead, mercury and arsenic are also considered trace elements despite their association with environmental pollution. These poisonous elements have always been found in nature, but only rarely have they been present at considerable concentrations. Today however, modern industrial practices have strained wide regions of land and many resources by loading dangerous amounts of toxins into the ecosystem (including poisonous trace elements as well as radioactive materials and toxic organic compounds). This can lead to widespread pollution as demonstrated by the following two examples.

Radioactive fallout from the Chernobyl nuclear reactor disaster was spread over a huge area extending over half of Europe. The production of acid rain, primarily in mid-Europe, has damaged forests and surrounding bodies of water, and has led to the creation of biologically dead lakes in northern

Europe (especially Sweden and Finland). As our soils (and therefore the plants and animals raised on them) are increasingly being exposed to toxins, a steady intensification of agricultural practices is leading to an increased depletion of trace elements. While nitrogenous fertilizers increase grain yield, soil fertility suffers due to a lack of the essential trace minerals. The rise of processing taking place in the food industry is contributing to a further decline of biologically important, quality food ingredients. This is especially apparent in fast-food products – hamburgers, for example. Unfortunately, many food products are diminishing in biological value. Even if food products leave the factory with nutritional content intact, the important nutrients are often lost during transport despite attempts to supplement foods with vitamins. In addition, these foods frequently contain considerable amounts of additives. Consumers have become overly concerned with the appearance and taste of commercial foods. To appease consumers, many manufacturers add vitamins and minerals to products to compensate for nutrients depleted in processing.

The result of conventional food processing is a deficiency of important substances. The risk of nutrient deficiency increases if you have a restrictive diet, a pre-existing nutrient deficiency, or if you are elderly. Due to the deficiency of nutrients in our food supply, we have extra nutritional requirements especially during:

- childhood growth, pregnancy and nursing periods
- performance-demanding situations, (perhaps secondary to chronic illness)
- recovery periods after illness or surgery (convalescence)
- illnesses that disable nutrient uptake from the small intestine
- periods of increased nutrient loss.

The consequences of deficient mineral intake (increased frequency of complaints and eventually serious illness) can sometimes take years to appear, as exemplified by the development of osteoporosis.

To study this area further, more than a few general facts are needed. A review of this field is especially important because many sources of information are available today. Many people seek nutritional counseling to help them understand their nutritional requirements. Most nutritional counselors rarely cover issues beyond calories, carbohydrates, protein and fat. Extra nutritional requirements are usually only considered for pregnant women, and in these cases only calcium ("for the bones") and iron ("for the blood") are recommended.

Some countries have addressed nutrient deficiency by supplementing their food supply with minerals. A successful and cost-effective trace element supplementation program is the iodization of table salt for the prevention of goiter. If the 90% decline in thyroid disease in Switzerland (where only iodized salt is available) were to be extended into (West) Germany, it would correspond to an annual savings of one-half billion US dollars. Similar progress achieved in the former East Germany was lost after reunification due to the introduction of "West German" salt (see Iodine chapter).

Trace minerals are an important component of soil and therefore have a role in gardening and farming practices. Conventional gardening books often describe and recommend various trace elements that are important to plants. In farming practice, salt stones are given to animals to compensate for trace element deficiencies found in the soil. Even the fields of veterinary medicine and sports medicine utilize knowledge of trace elements.

The safety of trace minerals is an important consideration. The potential to do harm exists in any medical intervention including trace mineral supplementation. The authors have attempted to educate the reader on the consequences of toxic mineral doses and the inappropriate use of trace minerals.

The public's perception of trace minerals is dependent on the way advertisers (and media) choose to portray them. It is understandable that advertisers target attention toward their own products rather than alternative or competing products. In doing so, scientific facts are eventually simplified and singled out to a great extent. The consumer is thereby presented with a limited, one-sided view. This type of advertising often gives the impression that a product can help almost anyone with almost any ailment. Many products sold this way are particularly confusing to the layperson.

Before reading the main sections of the book it may be useful to review the following terms: body content, daily requirement, and absorption rate.

"Body content" describes the quantity of the element found in an adult body of average weight (70 kg). For sodium, this would be 100 g and for potassium this would be 140 g. For cadmium, a relatively abundant but poisonous element, the body content of a 50 year old would be 15 mg (30 mg if this person is a smoker).

"Daily requirement" refers to the recommended daily intake of each element. For sodium, this would be 2-3 g (corresponding to 5 g of table salt) and for potassium this would be 3-4 g.

"Rate of absorption" signifies the fraction of the ingested amount that is taken up by the small intestine.

With American state medical exam (ECFMG) qualification and a keen interest in chemistry, Dr. Klaus-Georg Wenzel provides a unique overview of the trace elements. With a BDDT-N board certification in Naturopathic Medicine, and with a focus on nutritional medicine, Raymond Pataracchia

Trace Mineral	Body Content	Daily Requirement	Absorption Rate
Ca (Calcium)	1000 g	800-1200 mg	varies
Mg (Magnesium)	25-35 g	300-400 mg	25-75 %
Si (Silicon)	1 g	20-200 mg	1-4 %
Zn (Zinc)	2-4 g	15 mg	10-40 %
Fe (Iron)	4-5 g	10-15 mg	5-20 %
Mn (Manganese)	10-40 mg	3-5 mg	5-40 %
Cu (Copper)	80-100 mg	2-3 mg	often only 5 %
Mo (Molybdenum)	20 mg	50-250 µg	varies
Cr (Chromium)	2-6 mg	50-200 µg	1-25 %
I (Iodine)	10-30 mg	200 µg	100%
Se (Selenium)	10-30 mg	50-200 µg	50-100 %

provides a further comprehensive component to this book. This book is intended for medical professionals and non-professionals.

To review all aspects of trace elements would not be possible in this book, as it would require reference to an enormous collection of research literature. Due to the explosive growth of knowledge in this field, some parts of this book may already have been supplemented by new discoveries at the time of printing.

This book is organized for easy access to information. Trace minerals are described individually in Section 1. One-page summaries of trace minerals are provided on the first page of each chapter. The reader can also look up a specific disease or symptom by using the index at the back of the book. The reader will find that this book reads more like a story than a text book without losing sight of clinically important details.

Regarding unit measures: 1 µg = 1 mcg = 0.001 mg.

THE
INDIVIDUAL
MINERALS

SILVER

Latin: *Argentum* – chemical symbol **Ag**

Functions: none known

Therapeutic applications: astringent when applied externally
corrosive
enhances wound granulation
bactericide, disinfectant

Negative biological effects: possible inner organ damage and
"rheumatic-like" joint complaints
when ingested

Sources: silver-containing eye drops
dental amalgam (besides Hg and Sn)
photography paper

SILVER
An ancient remedy

Silver has been used as an external remedy for a long time. At low concentrations it acts as an astringent and also kills bacteria by reacting with bacterial proteins. At higher concentrations, such as in the lunar caustic form, it is corrosive. For prevention of gonococcal conjunctivitis (infection on the membranes of the eyeball and eyelid) in newborns, one drop of a 1-2% silver nitrate solution is administered into each eye. These drops are considered necessary because gonorrheal-type eye infections following birth can lead to blindness.

In the case where silver is taken up by the body and distributed by the blood, damage can occur to the inner organs in particular, and rheumatic complaints can also arise. These negative effects can be intensified by deficiencies in zinc and copper, which are antagonistic (act in opposition) to silver. A patient is described (she is a gold and silversmith) whose rheumatic condition had previously been treated unsuccessfully at several orthopedic clinics (see Section 2). A career change was not an option, so after a working diagnosis of silver excess was made, treatment led to symptom improvement and the patient remained active in her career.

The symptoms of silver poisoning are described in the literature as follows: rheumatic complaints in the muscles, ligaments, joints and spine; headaches; nausea; memory loss; anxiety; and rapid exhaustion. Overdoses of silver can cause, among other things, argyrosis conjunctivitis – permanent pigmentation of connective tissue (and eventually corneal tissue) due to silver deposition. This most often results from the administration of silver-containing eye drops.

At the beginning of the 20th century, circuses would present the "Blue man", who after 35 years of work in a silver mine, had accumulated silver deposits almost everywhere in his body, especially visible all over his skin.

Besides mercury and tin, dental amalgams (fillings) contain considerable amounts of silver.

Due to industrial waste, 2500 tonnes of silver were released into the environment worldwide in 1977. At the moment, environmental levels of silver do not pose a general risk to the public.

ALUMINUM

chemical symbol **Al**

Functions:

none known

Therapeutic applications:

antacids such as aluminum hydroxide bind to acids (the neutralizing effect relieves heartburn)

constituent in deodorants

Negative biological effects:

digestive problems including intestinal colic
constipation
appetite suppression
involved in Alzheimer's disease?

Sources:

pots, pans, aluminum foil and other cooking utensils made of aluminum, especially when heated and/or acid treated

deodorants
processed cheese
aluminum-rich water, especially water containing additives from treatment plants

Preventing toxicity:

supplements to diminish aluminum levels
• calcium, magnesium
• vitamins C and B6
• sulfur-containing amino acids
  (e.g. cysteine)

ALUMINUM

The malleable metal of limited medicinal use

As 8% of the earth's crust is aluminum, it is the most abundant metal on earth. It is found at (varying) low levels in plant and animal tissues, and is not considered essential for life.

Bauxite is the raw material from which aluminum is made. During its mining a high concentration of dust is released into the air which can lead to rare cases of lung disease (aluminum silicosis) among the workers.

Due to the varying aluminum content within the earth's soil, its concentration in water fluctuates accordingly. Some water treatment facilities use aluminum sulfate to precipitate turbid organic matter. The aluminum in your water supply adheres to hair surfaces. Performing hair mineral analysis when your water supply has high aluminum levels will artificially elevate levels.

External therapeutics such as alum and aluminum acetate are playing a dwindling role in the medical field. Aluminum-coated dressings are used for large wounds and burn surfaces. At high intakes, increased amounts of aluminum can be found in the brain, bones, muscles, kidneys, thyroid and lungs. This may lead to negative consequences.

Aluminum passing through the stomach and intestines is predominantly excreted in the stool. Usually only 1-3% of it is absorbed. The kidneys play the most important role in the excretion of absorbed aluminum. This process is only compromised when kidney function is greatly diminished, as in patients on kidney dialysis. Aluminum is implicated in the higher incidence of brain and bone damage occurring in kidney dialysis patients. This includes osteomalacia (bone softening) and encephalopathy, with the latter appearing during dialysis and regressing within 24 hours. Recent discoveries have suggested that the increased aluminum uptake by the brain in Alzheimer's is more likely a result as opposed to a cause of the disease.

Aluminum excretion is promoted by vitamin C and B6, sulfur-containing amino acids, and by the antagonistic effects of calcium and magnesium. If you have a high protein diet, the intestinal tract will likely absorb aluminum more readily.

ARSENIC

chemical symbol **As**

poisonous ☠

Functions:	none known – arsenic is toxic to cells
Therapeutic applications:	in out-of-date medications
Negative biological effects:	fatigue diarrhea and inflammation of the gastric mucosa increased hair loss skin pigmentation nerve damage – polyneuropathy
Sources:	combustion of coal insecticides, pesticides and plant preservatives (previously used regularly in vineyards) metal manufacturing glass production previously in wallpaper, paints and some medications
Factors that prevent toxicity:	selenium sulfur-containing amino acids (e.g. cysteine) vitamins C and E

ARSENIC

A fashionable poison of previous centuries

Arsenic is present practically everywhere in minute quantities, especially in smog and industrial emissions (therefore contributing to environmental pollution). Poisoning among vineyard workers exposed to pesticides was frequent in former times, as was poisoning among those exposed to arsenic-containing wallpaper and paint.

After being taken up by the body, arsenic binds to tissues and is stored on a long-term basis especially in the hair, skin, nails, kidneys and liver. This facilitates the development of cancer, particularly in the liver, bronchi and skin.

Arsenic is eliminated slowly by urine, stool, perspiration, breath (garlicky odor), and to a certain extent through nails and hair (where it can be reliably measured by hair mineral analysis).

Between 1990 and 1992, 3.6% of adults and 2.2% of children in Germany had urine arsenic values over 40 µg/L. Anything above this level poses a long-term health hazard.

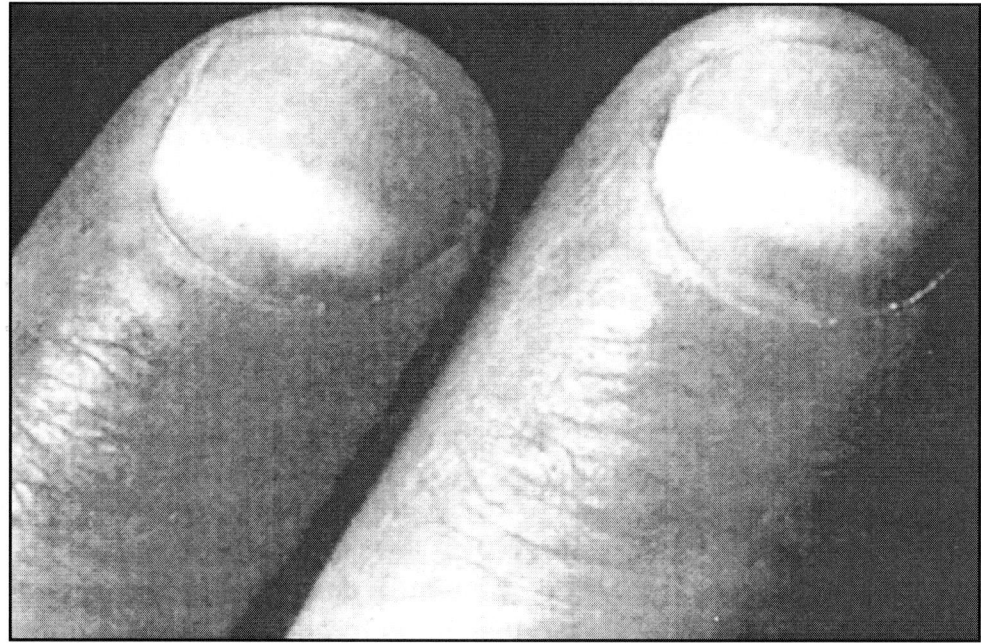

Mees' bands seen as a result of chronic arsenic poisoning

Arsenic is toxic in every form and acts, above all, as a capillary and enzymatic poison. After uptake through the air or intestinal tract, acute or chronic poisoning develops. Acute poisoning leads to nausea and vomiting, developing into massive intestinal tract inflammation with diarrhea two hours later. The water and salt loss from this can lead to shock, kidney failure, coma and respiratory paralysis. If the patient survives, permanent liver and kidney damage is common.

Chronic poisoning is caused predominantly by occupational exposure to arsenic-containing materials and leads to the following symptoms: increased hair loss; rashes (eczematous, pustulating, ulcerous) around the nose, skin folds and mucosa; dark gray skin pigmentation; wart-like skin eruptions, especially on the inner hands and soles of the feet; eventual skin cancer; white vertical stripes (Mees' bands) on fingernails; nerve damage (sensory motor polyneuropathy) and conjunctivitis of the eyes.

The ancient Greek, Roman and Germanic blacksmiths were all crippled. Since arsenic was melted with copper in the Bronze Age, the blacksmiths suffered from chronic arsenic poisoning which led to paralysis.

In Europe, occupational illnesses due to arsenic exposure are covered by health insurance and are compensated for by wage indemnity programs.

Small quantities of arsenic intake, such as from the consumption of seafood (which contains relatively large amounts of arsenic due to water pollution and natural weathering of rock), will not lead to poisoning due to the excretory functions of the liver and kidneys.

The toxic dose of arsenic lies between 10-50 mg. For the time being, the WHO currently considers the safe tolerance level for adults to be 1 mg of arsenic per week.

Arsenic was often used as a murder poison in the Middle Ages. Some individuals seem to have killed up to 500 people with it! It became a "fashionable" way to murder. Nowadays, arsenic can easily be detected years after death (especially in hair). During some periods in the Middle Ages, there was even a belief that small quantities of arsenic improved the diet and lead to fuller figures and better complexions among pale women. It was used among horse breeders, and in Tyrol (in northern Italy). Many lumberjacks and mountain climbers took it to boost their performance. These so-called "arsenic eaters" could build up a tolerance for arsenic in the range of four times the toxic dosage. Today, these preparations (known as "Fowler's drops" or "Asian pills") are unthinkable.

In countries like Pakistan, millions of people have high arsenic concentrations in their drinking water. According to the UNO, 20,000 people die every year in Pakistan due to arsenic poisoning. Some people are dying of cancer secondary to long-term (up to 30 years) arsenic exposure.

According to the WHO-recommendation in Europe, drinking water is allowed to contain a maximum of 10 μg/L of arsenic. When President George W. Bush became president in the US, he canceled an arsenic-reducing law for drinking water. In the US, arsenic sources, in addition to natural sources, include chemicals used in plant and wood preservatives and the mining industry.

GOLD

Latin: *Aurum* – chemical symbol **Au**

Functions: none known

Therapeutic applications: chronic polyarthritis
psoriatic arthritis
therapeutic dosages of 5-50 mg per day

radioactive gold (Au-198) is used for radiation of tumors

Negative biological effects: possible inner organ damage and "rheumatic" complaints upon intake

Sources: medications
frequent exposure to and processing of gold

GOLD

Precious or not?

As a noble metal, gold is chemically resistant. For this reason, and for the ease with which it is processed, gold is widely used in dentistry and jewelry making. Since gold is non-corrosive and conducts electricity well, it is used in the electrical industry for high-end switches and contact points.

Since 1927, gold compounds have been used to treat chronic polyarthritis. 30% of patients experience significant side effects because gold builds up in tissues over time and acts as a capillary poison. Slate-gray to blue-violet skin pigmentations can develop, especially on areas exposed to light. In addition, inflammation can occur to mucous membranes in the mouth, and gold deposits can form in the corneas. Associated bone marrow damage can lead to serious changes in blood formation, up to and including aplastic anemia.

Radioactive gold (Au-198) emits beta and gamma rays and is used for the radiation of certain tumors. It is stored in the liver and spleen and is excreted very slowly in stool and urine.

The rheumatic complaints of a a gold- and silver-smith are described in the silver section, as well as in the laboratory chapter.

BORON

chemical symbol **B**

Normal daily requirement: 1-2 mg
(therapeutic doses up to 3 mg)

Functions: immune system
membrane stability, cell division
calcium and vitamin regulation

Therapeutic applications: allergies
skin conditions
rheumatism and gout
weakened immune functions, including cancer
osteoporosis (calcium sparing function)

Negative biological effects: upon excessive intake:
- stomach and intestinal cramps
- damage to bone marrow, liver, kidneys,
- lungs and brain

Sources: dates, poppy seeds, dandelion, turnips, beets, legumes, red wine

overdoses are possible from boron compounds in preservatives, fertilizers and cleaning products

Note: boron supports the uptake of vitamin C, flavonoids and sulfur-containing amino acids

uptake of boron is hindered or prevented by: chlorine, chlorinated hydrocarbons, wood varnish and high percentage alcohol

BORON
The immune booster

Boron was used as a food preservative in the form of Borax. Since it is almost fully absorbed by the intestine, builds up in the body when taken in large amounts, and is excreted slowly, negative effects can be recognized fairly quickly. Poisoning symptoms include: stomach and intestinal cramps including vomiting and diarrhea; damage to lungs, liver, kidneys and bone marrow; and eventual brain injury including confusion, dizziness and depression.

The positive effects of boron, especially its complex binding capabilities, have been overlooked. Boron is important for proper functioning of the immune system, cellular metabolism (including cell division and repair), as well as calcium and vitamin regulation. It is especially important in connection with calcium and flavonoids to maintain the structure and elasticity of cell walls and membranes.

Insufficient intake of boron leads to an increased frequency of allergy symptoms (including hay fever), abnormal skin conditions, and diminished performance of the immune system, heart and various other organs.

The high boron content in bones is important for blood formation and immune functions of the bone marrow. The reduced levels of boron in elderly people could play a role in the development of osteoporosis. Sufficient boron content seems to be important for the action of estrogen and testosterone – especially when these hormones diminish during and after menopause.

Boron deficiency is perpetuated by chlorinated water, chlorinated hydrocarbons such as wood varnishes and certain antibiotics, and also by strong alcohols. Boron deficiency increases cell wall breakage, facilitating the entrance of poisons and viruses. This seems to play a role in dying forests. Heavily damaged trees in the Black Forest recuperated after soils were supplemented with boron. For plants, boron also plays a role in photosynthesis.

BARIUM

chemical symbol **Ba**

Functions:

none known
soluble salts are poisonous

Therapeutic applications:

its insoluble compounds are used in the medical field to create contrast for X-rays

Negative biological effects:

upon intake of soluble salts:
- vomiting and diarrhea
- nausea
- disruption of cardiac rhythm, including ventricular fibrillation

Sources:

plant pesticides
fur removal agents
heavy spar

BARIUM

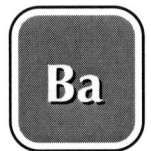

An X-ray contrast element

Barium belongs to the alkaline earth metals along with magnesium, calcium and strontium.

In nature, barium is found in heavy spar and barites of minerals and ores. Exposure to dust by working in these environments can lead to lung problems.

Because barium has a high atomic mass, it is used in the insoluble and non-toxic form of barium sulfate to achieve better contrast in x-rays of the stomach and intestinal tract.

Only soluble barium salts are poisonous. They cause smooth muscle spasms, vomiting, stomach aches, diarrhea, nausea and decreased blood pressure. They also lead to significant disruptions in cardiac rhythm, including ventricular fibrillation (which is eventually fatal).

Barium compounds are used in rat and mouse poisons, pesticides and fur removal agents.

BERYLLIUM

chemical symbol **Be**

poisonous ☠

Functions:

none known – poisonous trace element

Therapeutic applications:

Negative biological effects:

poisoning symptoms:
- fever, coughing
- conjunctivitis
- erythemia and eczema
- stomach ulcers
- damage to the lungs, heart, liver, bones and brain

Sources:

inner coating of fluorescent tubes
metal processing industry
electrical industry
high tech ceramics

BERYLLIUM

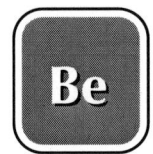

A rare toxic element

Beryllium is a rare element – a very hard metal, which forms alloys with a variety of other metals. Highly permeable to X-rays, it is used in the ray emission window of X-ray tubes.

Beryllium and its compounds can enter the body primarily in the form of dust and vapors. At first, this results in a feverish illness that progresses into severe lung and heart damage. This overall poisoning effect also involves kidney, liver, bone marrow and central nervous system damage. Severe beryllium poisoning may lead to death by respiratory paralysis.

Beryllium deposits in the bones lead to skeletal structure changes known as beryllium-arthralgia.

Occupational exposure to beryllium occurs particularly in the fields of high-tech ceramics, electronics, metal processing, aerospace and nuclear technology. About 5% of the workers in these fields develop lung disease, which appears to have a genetic component and does not affect all individuals in the same manner. In Europe, damages due to occupational beryllium exposure are covered by health insurance and are compensated for by wage indemnity programs.

Cuts from broken, beryllium-coated fluorescent tubes can happen to anyone. These wounds are dangerous and heal very slowly (forming granulomas, fistulas and keloids).

BISMUTH

chemical symbol **Bi**

Functions: not known

Therapeutic applications: used externally for the treatment of wounds and for mucosal inflammation

Negative biological effects: stomatitis

discoloration and eventual inflammation of the gums and tongue

in rare cases, disturbance of brain function

Sources: bismuth preparations
synthetic jewels

BISMUTH

The stomach ulcer remedy

Bismuth has been used for a long time in various compounds for medical purposes. Ointments (mostly containing about 10% bismuth) are used externally to treat wounds and eczema, acting as astringents and antihydrotics (prevents sweating). In tablet form, daily bismuth dosages of 300 mg are used to treat gastrointestinal conditions.

Lately, bismuth has been used to relieve stomach ulcers. *Helicobacter pylori* plays a significant role in chronic gastric mucosal inflammation. Bismuth can effectively inhibit this bacterium. In addition, it forms a protective coating over the gastric mucosa by reacting with bacterial proteins in the stomach's acidic environment.

Previously, bismuth was used to treat syphilis and parasitic infections. In the meantime, more effective options have been developed.

Bismuth was also known to cause damage when it was injected intramuscularly and intravenously ("Bismuth-flu"). In tablet form, it is not recommended to take bismuth preparations over long periods of time nor in high dosages since they can be toxic. A temporary blue-black discoloration of the tongue is considered normal. Similar to other heavy metals, however, bismuth can cause a gray-blue edge along the gums following long-term use. This should be interpreted as a warning symptom. As poisoning progresses, the tongue also becomes inflamed.

About 20 years ago, cases appeared in France and Australia in which patients temporarily experienced disturbances in brain function with daily bismuth dosages over 1.5 g. These patients had a colostomy and were taking 5-15 g of bismuth daily over long periods of time to eliminate odors. Hallucinations, anxiety attacks, speech and concentration disturbances, as well as occasional cases of epileptic seizures, coma and death occurred.

As a precaution, pregnant women or anyone with kidney disease should avoid bismuth.

BROMINE

chemical symbol **Br**

Functions: not known

Therapeutic applications: previously used in sedatives
and to treat epilepsy

Negative biological effects: acne, rashes
allergies, hyperhidrosis (excessive sweating)
lung damage
bromine addiction
bromism

Sources: medications
film and photo industry
dyes and solvents

BROMINE

The element that competes with chlorine

Bromine belongs to the halogens along with chlorine, iodine and fluorine. This explains the antagonism often seen between these elements in terms of their biological function.

Upon uptake by the body, bromine salts displace chlorine salts. If more than 10% of serum chloride is replaced by bromide, brain function is disrupted resulting in sleeplessness, diminished memory and decreased concentration. Replacing 20-30% of the body's serum chloride results in hallucinations, confusion, speech disruptions, and a decline in general well-being.

Like iodine, bromine is stored in the thyroid gland.

Since the kidneys cannot distinguish between bromide and chloride, the effectiveness of bromide is strongly dependent on table salt (sodium chloride) intake.

The bromine compounds previously applied as sedatives and to treat epilepsy are hardly in use today due to the availability of safer, more effective medications. Furthermore, a type of bromine dependency can result from taking these compounds.

Rashes with blister formations have been reported as allergic reactions among patients sensitive to bromine. Acne can also result among highly sensitive individuals. Inhalation of elemental bromine vapors can irritate and damage mucosal tissues of the lungs and respiratory tract.

Silver bromide is used to make copy paper and film due to its light sensitivity.

CALCIUM

chemical symbol **Ca**

essential for life

Normal daily requirement:	children and adults 800-1200 mg pregnant and nursing women 1400 mg infants 250-500 mg after menopause 1500 mg
Functions:	development of bones and teeth nerve and muscle function, including cardiac muscle
Therapeutic applications:	pregnancy and nursing periods osteoporosis (bone decalcification) allergies (as injections) nervousness, sleep disorders
Sources:	milk and dairy products such as cheese and yogurt fish whole grain breads
Note:	calcium uptake is promoted by: • vitamins D, C, A • gastric acid calcium uptake is hindered by: • the formation of insoluble compounds with phosphate (in soft drinks, sausages and processed cheese) and phytate (in whole grain products and cereals) • oxalic acid (especially in rhubarb) • excess fat

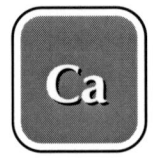

CALCIUM
Not just for the bones

Calcium is indispensable for the strength and development of bones and teeth. Even though these contain the majority of the body's calcium (about 1 kg in an adult), calcium is also essential in other areas.

Calcium is important for the transmission of impulses in nerve and muscle cells, including cardiac muscle cells. Calcium's significance to the structure and function of cellular membranes also applies to many other cells. It plays a role in allergic and inflammatory reactions (hence one of its therapeutic uses) as well as in blood clotting. Blood is mixed with calcium solutions during laboratory analyses to prevent it from coagulating.

Due to calcium's important roles in the body, an intricate regulatory mechanism exists between it and vitamin D (which increases intestinal absorption of calcium when in high demand), and with calcitonin and parathyroid hormone. Long term intake of medications such as cortisone and "water pills" (diuretics) influence this regulation by increasing calcium excretion. Mobilizing calcium deposits in bone can easily compensate for short-term calcium deficiencies. However, long-term calcium deficiency does lead to problems.

Early folk medicine brought up the saying "every child costs its mother one tooth" (about 20 g of calcium is supplied by a mother to her developing child, therefore extra calcium intake is recommended to pregnant women). It is a good idea to take newborns outdoors on a daily basis to promote the formation of vitamin D. It was commonly thought that a few minutes of light (UV ray) exposure, even on overcast days, was enough to form sufficient vitamin D in skin cells. However, research suggests that vitamin D deficiency in adults and children is more common than we realize. Many people also become calcium-deficient by taking calcium without vitamin D. Optimal doses of vitamin D (for an adult) are in the range of 1000 IU per day. People who are not exposed to ultraviolet rays over long periods of time due to illness or working conditions cannot synthesize adequate amounts of vitamin D. This causes a disruption of calcium regulation and in severe instances, may lead to rickets. Some daily sun exposure will help to maintain vitamin D levels. Excessive sun tanning is not necessary for vitamin D formation.

Osteoporosis (see also the Fluorine chapter) is a common disease affecting both women and men. A low calcium diet over several decades is a significant factor in the development of osteoporosis. This has also been attributed to changes in the population's eating habits over the last few decades. Currently, the typical diet contains too little calcium in relation to its caloric value due to the altering and processing of foods. Female sex hormones (especially estrogen) slow calcium excretion from the kidneys. When estrogen levels drop as women enter menopause, the rate of calcium excretion increases. The American Osteoporosis Association recommends that women take (on a long-time basis) 1000 mg per day of calcium before menopause and 1500 mg per day after menopause. The most important time for women to ensure adequate calcium intake is before menarche as bone calcium absorption/deposition is approximately five times that during adulthood.

In 1992, a German medical journal reported a New Zealand study to monitor the effect of calcium supplementation in menopausal women. In a randomized and placebo-controlled study, a statistically significant decrease in bone density loss was observed among women who took an extra 1000 mg of calcium daily over a two year period.

There is new scientific data that strontium downregulates the osteoclast cells and stimulates the new bone-building osteoblast cells. This is therefore under investigation for osteoporosis treatment.

Not many people are aware that bones take up an increased amount of other elements during calcium deficiency. Besides strontium (and other alkaline earth metals such as barium), heavy metals like lead and cadmium are also absorbed more strongly. Therefore, elevated lead levels in the environment can exacerbate problems associated with calcium deficiency. Radioactive strontium-90, released by atomic weapon tests and nuclear reactor accidents, is highly absorbed by the bones. Taking in extra calcium can reduce this heavy metal deposition. Likewise, additional iodine (in the form of tablets, as should be found in nuclear emergency shelters) will hinder the uptake of radioactive iodine by the thyroid gland.

Proper intestinal uptake of calcium depends greatly on digestive enzymes (especially those secreted by the pancreas) as well as adequate gastric acid. Good intestinal bacterial activity is also very important. This can sometimes be improved by supplementing with *Lactobacillus acidophilus*.

When cells or cellular membranes take up increased amounts of calcium (oxygen-depleted heart or brain cells for example), aberrant metabolic reactions, including cell death, can result. Calcium antagonism is an important principle behind various heart, brain and blood vessel (including migraine) medications. Calcium antagonists include not only these medicines, but also magnesium ("the natural calcium antagonist") and, to some extent, zinc.

This illustrates that even a common mineral such as calcium should not be viewed in isolation from other elements in the body.

Reasons for calcium deficiency include:

1. Low intake of calcium-rich products (especially milk, dairy products and vegetables). This occurs particularly among women on calorie-restricted diets.

2. Dietary additives which hinder calcium absorption:
   - phosphate in soft drinks, sausages and processed cheese;
   - phytate, especially in cereal bran. However, the phytase enzyme found in cereals normally frees minerals bound to phytate (i.e. calcium, iron, magnesium, zinc) during dough processing;
   - oxalic acid in spinach, rhubarb, black tea and cocoa.

3. Calcium losses due to cooking practices (lengthy cooking or soaking allows calcium to escape into the surrounding water). Calcium loss can also occur through the kidneys due to excessive alcohol, nicotine or caffeine intake. Alcohol disrupts vitamin D metabolism.

Prolonged low calcium levels lead to changes in hair, skin and nails. Muscle tetany can also occur when calcium is low. Cataracts, which can eventually lead to blindness, may also develop under low calcium conditions.

Calcium acts synergistically with magnesium and phosphorous/phosphate. It is therefore recommended to take calcium, phosphorous, and magnesium in relative ratios of 1 : 1(-1.5) : 0.5 parts, respectively.

70-90% of calcium secretion takes place via the intestinal tract, mainly due to the rich supply of digestive juices.

Calcium intake above the recommended daily dosage, such as for the reduction of allergic reactions, will only lead to elevated blood calcium levels for relatively short periods of time. This does not lead to "calcification", as is often feared.

Problems involving elevated calcium levels are rare and predominantly involve people with kidney disease, other rare illness, or vitamin D poisoning which is rare (secondary to eating polar bear liver or excessive amounts of cod liver oil).

CADMIUM

chemical symbol **Cd**

poisonous ☠

Functions:	none – very poisonous!
Therapeutic applications:	none
Poisoning symptoms:	kidney damage, high blood pressure loss of appetite and sense of smell disrupts calcium metabolism bone and joint pain heart and blood vessel damage
Sources:	cigarette smoke! contaminated seafood automobile emissions food coloring cadmium batteries
Factors that protect against cadmium:	zinc, selenium, calcium, copper sulfur-containing amino acids sulfur foods, vitamin C, and B6

CADMIUM

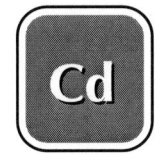

The poisonous pretty yellow pigment

Cadmium is a toxin that can hardly be removed from the environment. It is only released into the air through human activity. It has become the most abundant poisonous trace element besides lead. Since the beginning of the 20th century, cadmium production has increased by a factor of 1000 through industrialization!

In theory, this cadmium will end up in the atmosphere sooner or later. It is estimated that every year in Germany alone, 83 tonnes of cadmium are released into the air, 62 tonnes into the waters, and 124 tonnes in the waste of industries and residences.

Main producers are the iron and steel industry, followed by the combustion of coal and oil by homes, industrial plants, power stations, and garbage incinerators. This illustrates the importance of emission filters in chimneys. An additional environmental risk arises due to the cadmium content of many phosphate fertilizers and pesticides.

Cadmium is probably best known as a pigment. In the military, objects painted with a green cadmium pigment have the same light and infrared reflections as grass and leaves, making them unnoticeable on aerial photographs.

The largest amount (about 50% of total cadmium production) is manufactured into cadmium alloys, including metal solder. Cadmium is also used for battery production, PVC plastic stabilization, rust protection, glass production, galvanizing, as well as neutron deceleration in nuclear reactors.

Considerable amounts are found in cigarette smoke! The average person inhales about 0.4 µg of cadmium from smoke and consumes about 30 µg in their food and drinking water (but twice as much if the food was grown in the proximity of a metal processing plant!). 15 cigarettes provide about 2 µg, 50% of which is absorbed by the lungs. Only 5% is absorbed by the intestinal tract, providing some protection to non-smokers.

Since only 1 µg can be excreted per day, the remainder is deposited in the liver and kidneys. Cadmium's half-life is between 10 and 30 years (the time it takes to excrete half of a particular amount of cadmium from the body). This creates the possibility of cumulative poisoning. It is practically impossible to have a completely cadmium-free diet.

While newborns hardly have any cadmium in their systems, a 50 year old adult has about 15 mg (30 mg if he or she is a smoker!).

Approximately one third of the total cadmium content in the human body is stored in the kidneys. The kidneys are the most sensitive to cadmium poisoning, which can result in high blood pressure.

The harmful effects of cadmium are accentuated by zinc deficiency, since cells take up increased amounts of cadmium under these circumstances. In the periodic table of elements, cadmium is found directly below zinc, and one row beneath that is mercury!

The first symptom of kidney damage is an increased excretion of blood into the urine (proteinuria). Proteinuria (excess protein in the urine) increases with the amount of cadmium found in the body and kidneys.

Cadmium causes skeletal damage by impairing calcium/phosphate metabolism (causing bladder stone formation), impairing vitamin D metabolism, and compromising the zinc-containing alkaline phosphatase enzyme.

Cadmium disrupts the metabolism of other elements – zinc and copper in particular. Zinc deficiency due to chronic cadmium poisoning leads to a decrease and possibly abolishment of smell and taste senses. Besides this, cadmium disrupts acid/base regulation (with acidosis) and hinders the intestinal absorption of iron.

Along with lead, it weakens the immune system. An animal experiment showed that this effect could be counteracted to some extent by vitamin C supplementation.

Occupational cadmium poisoning is covered under health insurance plans in Germany, and is compensated for by wage indemnity programs.

A particularly sad example of environmental cadmium pollution is an illness that arose in the Japanese province of Toyama. Due to the painful cries of affected patients, it was named Itai-Itai disease. This disease primarily affected women who had several children and who lived in this area over many decades. Due to the cadmium-polluted waste water of a local zinc mine, drinking water and rice (their staple food) fields became contaminated, leading to cadmium poisoning. This led to atrophy and decalcification of practically all bones in the skeletal system, causing a great deal of pain. These patients shrank about 30 cm in height. Even the slightest shaking movements could lead to fractures, such as rib fractures upon coughing. One unfortunate victim had 72 breaks, 28 of which were rib fractures. Until 1968, 114 women and five men died, mostly due to kidney failure or infections. In retrospect, deficiencies in calcium, vitamin D and protein likely played roles in this illness.

The use of cadmium alloys for water and food containers has been banned since 1950. Food stored in these types of containers caused serious disease symptoms. Similar to acute food poisoning, gastrointestinal complaints occurred along with nausea, vomiting and diarrhea. Muscle cramps and increased salivation followed. Disruptions in fluid regulation led to circulatory system shock, kidney failure and liver damage. In some cases, this led to death within 1-2 weeks.

Acute cadmium poisoning can occur among workers who melt cadmium-containing alloys and inadvertently inhale the vapors. This causes inflammation of the airways and lungs (and sometimes fatal lung edema) as well as general toxicity symptoms (chest pains, diarrhea, headaches, dizziness and fever). Chelating agents are used to treat cadmium poisoning. These compounds bind to cadmium and allow it to be excreted. However, this does put stress on the kidneys as they are temporarily exposed to increased amounts of cadmium.

Vitamin C, B6, E, selenium and zinc help to counteract cadmium toxicity.

In light of the harmful effects of cadmium, a general goal should be to minimize its use and thereby prevent its release into the atmosphere. This can be accomplished by:
- minimizing the production and processing of cadmium by replacing it with non-toxic elements;
- decreasing the use of materials that pose a risk to the environment, so that people are exposed to them as little as possible by way of air, water and food. Phosphate fertilizers and sludge from sewage treatment facilities contain a high amount of cadmium and should no longer be used in agriculture;
- garbage incinerators and power plants or factories burning fossil fuels should install emission filters. The steel industry drastically reduced cadmium emissions after employing filters;
- diminishing the cadmium content of soils by cultivating maize (which extracts cadmium from the soil), adding lime (which immobilizes cadmium), and performing soil exchanges.

While good quality spring water only contains 0.05-0.15 µg of cadmium per liter, ground water in the vicinity of sewage treatment facility sludge or waste water deposits can contain 4-16 µg/L. Industrial waste water contains 100-1000 µg/L. Problematic water leaks from deposits are now thankfully directed to water treatment facilities. This filters out 50-90% of the cadmium, lessening the risk of ground water contamination. However, sludge should no longer be used as a fertilizer due to the risk it poses to ground water. Even though most rivers in Germany pass the drinking water limit of 6 µg/L, their sediment contains much higher concentrations of cadmium. In polluted rivers this can range from 30-400 mg/kg, compared to 1 mg/kg in clean rivers. In the end, it all goes out to the ocean!

CHLORINE

chemical symbol Cl

Daily requirement:

3-5 g for adults

Functions:

water regulation (together with sodium)
gastric acid

Therapeutic applications:

used to treat these deficiency symptoms:
- inadequate gastric acid
- poor digestion
- muscle weakness

Sources:

foods containing salt, such as:
cheese, sausages and fish

CHLORINE

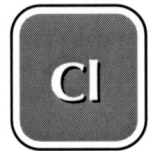

The gastric acid element

The body of an adult contains about 80 g of chlorine. It is primarily found with sodium and is important for water regulation and for the distribution of fluids within tissues.

Specialized acid-resistant mucosal cells utilize chloride to produce gastric acid. Hot spices, caffeine, alcohol, fried foods and histamine can enhance this action.

In principle, elevated chlorine levels can only be possible with excessive salt intake. This can be significant in the development of high blood pressure.

Surplus amounts are excreted by the urinary system.

The normal daily requirement of 3-5 g chlorine (in the form of chloride) is easily obtained from the diet.

Chloride deficiencies can develop as a result of prolonged vomiting or diarrhea.

Chloride losses of 50% can disrupt water regulation enough to cause life-threatening cases of edema within body tissues. This is especially worrisome if it occurs within the brain. Excessive sweating (such as during athletic activities) can diminish muscular performance. It is recommended to take in adequate amounts of salt under these circumstances.

COBALT

chemical symbol **Co**

Functions:

central atom of vitamin B12

daily requirement of vitamin B12 is 5 μg

Therapeutic applications:

vitamin B12 deficiency
(known as pernicious anemia)

also, generally for:
- anemia
- nerve damage
- vascular diseases

Negative biological effects:

none known, even with excessive vitamin B12 intake

problems only arise with inorganic cobalt compounds and with radioactive cobalt

Sources:

vitamin B12 is found predominantly in animal products, therefore deficiencies are relatively common among strict vegetarians

cobalt is released into the environment through emission gases and by cement, glass and metal industries

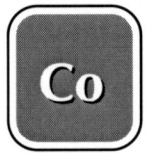

COBALT
The vitamin B12 element

The intensely red-colored vitamin B12 is the only vitamin with an inorganic component – it contains 4.5% cobalt bound to its complex.

About 1-10 mg of cobalt is found in the adult body, especially in the kidneys.

Vitamin B12 is utilized by many enzymes and is therefore required in all body cells. Presently known as the most effective biocatalyst, it is only required in daily amounts of 5-10 µg. If the stomach does not produce the intrinsic factor required to absorb vitamin B12, pernicious anemia will result. This can be accompanied by serious nerve damage (starting with sensory disturbances and eventually leading to paralysis). Up until 1926, 6,000 people – for example the mother of biochemist and Nobel Laurate Linus Pauling – died of this disease in the US alone! The role of the liver in B12 transport protein production was unknown in 1947. At that time, it was only known that some factor (vitamin B12) stored in the liver was helping to alleviate the symptoms of the disease.

Aside from its use as a B12 component, few other physiological roles involve cobalt. Experiments have shown that cobalt can replace zinc as a component of certain enzymes. It also influences the uptake of iodine in the thyroid gland and thereby reduces the formation of goiters.

Cobalt deficiencies among humans have not been documented, but they have been reported in animals grazing on cobalt-poor soils in Denmark, Australia and the US. A strong correlation between cobalt and vitamin B12 content in foods does not exist.

Excessive cobalt consumption (very rare) can lead to the following negative effects: loss of appetite, nausea, weight loss, enlargement of the thyroid gland and hypotony. Similar to other heavy metals it can cause nerve damage in the ears accompanied by ringing (tinnitus).

In certain industrial environments, inhalation of fine cobalt dust can lead to serious lung damage.

The radioactive isotope cobalt-60 arises as a result of nuclear reactions and is an unpleasant component of nuclear fall-out. Co-60 is used therapeutically for the radiation of deep tumors. More information about radioactive isotopes is found in Appendix 2.

CHROMIUM

chemical symbol **Cr**

recognized as an essential element in 1959

Normal daily requirement:
0.05-0.2 mg
up to 0.5 mg for therapeutic uses
(intestinal absorption 1-25%)

Functions:
as a component of glucose tolerance
factor (GTF), chromium is required to
activate insulin's regulation of blood sugar

thyroid function and fat metabolism

nucleic acid metabolism and synthesis

Therapeutic applications:
disturbances in sugar metabolism
cataracts and corneal damage
chronic infections

Negative biological effects:
almost exclusively associated
with chromium salts

Sources:
whole grain products (wheat germ)
corn, cheese, beer yeast, meat,
vegetables, potatoes

Note:
chromium can be released from heated pots
and pans or cooking utensils

cement and metal manufacturing industries
are main sources of environmental chromium
pollution

CHROMIUM

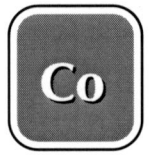

The sugar-regulating element

Chromium has been recognized as an essential trace element since 1959. The adult body contains about 2-6 mg of chromium. In humans, it is found in the form of a chromium-III complex.

The intestinal tract absorbs only 1-3% of chromium obtained from the diet in its salt form. Chromium is best absorbed (10-25%) when bound in an organic compound, such as the glucose tolerance factor (GTF) found in yeast, liver and meat. Published data describing the optimal daily intake of chromium indicate a range of between 0.05 and 0.2 mg. Excretion of chromium occurs primarily via the kidneys. Since sweat contains about ten times more chromium than blood serum, perspiration can increase the concentration of chromium measured in hair mineral analysis. Therefore, although an elevated chromium value in hair mineral analysis can be a sign of a high chromium intake (hardly possible by regular nutrition), it may also be due to perspiration. Excretion in diabetics is two to four times greater than in healthy individuals.

Chromium is important for thyroid function and sugar, amino acid, fat and nucleic acid metabolism. It is a component of the glucose tolerance factor (GTF) and the chromium-containing oligopeptide chromodulin, both of which activate the action of insulin to regulate blood sugar. Insulin is a pancreatic hormone that lowers blood sugar (glucose) levels by promoting its conversion into a storage form (glycogen) and by allowing cells to utilize blood sugar. Chromium deficiency is associated with elevated blood sugar levels (diabetes) as well as with low blood sugar levels (hypoglycemia).

Aside from its role in blood sugar regulation, chromium has also been reported to cause mild cholesterol lowering, anabolic effects, elevated sperm counts, and improved response to antidepressant treatment.

The salts derived from chromium-III are barely absorbed by the intestinal tract. On the other hand, chromium-VI compounds, found mainly in synthetic chemicals, are readily absorbed, relatively poisonous and promote allergic reactions. Even the chromium found in some dental cements can induce allergies.

Chromium poisoning, which develops primarily through inhalation or contact with skin or mucous membranes can present the following symptoms: eczema, ulcers, lung irritation (chromium silicosis), cancer, and asthma.

Occupational chromium poisoning is covered by wage indemnity programs and is compensated for by insurance in Europe.

COPPER

Latin: *Cuprum* – chemical symbol **Cu**

recognized as an **essential element** in 1928

Normal daily requirement:
children 0.4-2.5 mg, adults 2-4 mg
intestinal uptake often only 5%
Note: The therapeutic dosage lies within the
daily requirement range; greater quantities
over a longer term can lead to over-dosage.

Functions:
component of several enzymes,
especially superoxide dismutase (SOD) and
monoamine oxidase (MAO)

Copper is so important to the body that it has
its own blood transport protein, ceruloplasmin.
Failure to inherit the gene for this protein gives
rise to Wilson's disease.

Therapeutic applications:
blood formation (red and white blood cells)

color and elasticity of skin, hair and
connective tissue (therefore important for
growth and repair)

rheumatism

Copper is important for the brain, but
overdoses can be disruptive. MAO inhibitors
are prescribed for depression, anxiety and
Parkinson's disease.

Negative biological effects:
possible results of long term high-dose-intake:
• inner organ damage
• zinc deficiency due to antagonism

Sources:
like iron, copper is found in meat, fish, vegetables,
legumes, whole grains and nuts

released from copper water pipes, especially
during ion exchange treatment

COPPER
The element important for skin, hair, and more

Copper has been scientifically recognized as an essential trace element since 1928. An adult body contains 80-100 mg of copper. Quantitatively, it is the most significant element in the human body after iron and zinc. Only 5% of total body copper is found in the blood. Copper tends to concentrate in the liver at a level of 6.6 mg/kg of tissue, while the brain has 5.4, the heart 3.9, the kidneys 2.9, the spleen 1.2, muscles 0.9 and skin 0.7 mg/kg. Blood plasma of a healthy individual will carry about 1 mg/L.

Copper is important in the formation of red and white blood cells. It promotes the absorption of iron from the intestines. Several proteins containing copper are oxidizers.

A particularly important and well-known example of copper's function is its presence in superoxide dismutase, which offers protection from free radicals (reactive atoms that destroy cell components). Copper is also found in most antibodies and is therefore important for immune system function.

Other copper-bound enzymes include: ceruloplasmin (ferro-oxidase I), ferro-oxidase II, cytochrome-c-oxidase, amino-oxidase, dopamine-beta-hydroxylase, and tyrosinase.

Ceruloplasmin contains 8 copper atoms per molecule and has a variety of functions. It transports copper, oxidizes amines (e.g. catecholamines, serotonin), oxidizes ascorbic acid, and plays an important role in iron metabolism. Copper deficiency can therefore lead to symptoms of iron deficiency even if sufficient iron stores are present in the liver.

Cytochrome oxidase regulates the last and irreversible step of the electron transport chain in mitochondria and is thus an essential enzyme for cellular respiration. By compromising this action, a deficiency in copper can lead to decreased muscle performance and sluggish brain function.

Lysine monooxygenase is a monoamine oxidase. It is especially important in connective tissue to form cross linkages between the peptide chains of collagen and elastin.

Copper is also important for connective tissue regulation, especially for the formation of elastin. Elastin is responsible for maintaining the smoothness and elasticity of skin and it facilitates wound healing. Accordingly, copper deficiency is associated with chemical and physical changes in the skin and hair. Hair loses its color and becomes coarse (in extreme cases, it falls out).

Since copper is relatively abundant in food and water, deficiencies are rare. Usually only 5% of copper obtained from the diet is absorbed, but absorption is increased during periods of higher demand (such as during childhood growth). Adequate amounts of gastric acid are beneficial for absorption. Copper can also be taken up through skin. When skin is damaged, as in cases of eczema, absorption can increase 60 to 70-fold.

Excretion occurs primarily through bile, thereby passing through the intestines. The kidneys excrete very little copper.

Copper is poisonous in larger amounts. Bacteria and other microorganisms are especially sensitive to this and are quickly killed in copper containers (this is why flowers are preserved well in copper vases). In humans, elevated copper levels irritate mucous membranes and disrupt intestinal flora. However, this occurs almost only in cases of acute poisoning. In some instances irritation is strong enough to induce vomiting, which helps to hinder the onset of poisoning.

Long-term overdoses due to copper-rich drinking water led to the deaths of several children in southern Germany some time ago, as well as on some Native reserves in the US. Today, many older homes have copper water pipes that allow copper to accumulate in the standing water overnight. The relatively high copper levels found in morning tap water decrease throughout the day as standing water is replaced by a fresh public water supply.

The release of copper from water pipes is enhanced by the use of decalcifiers, which function as ion exchangers – an often forgotten side effect. For this reason, sodium hydroxide, lye, or acid binders such as phosphate or silicate preparations, are often added to water automatically (see Section 2 on page 130).

Copper pots and pans are now coated with another metal to avoid the release of copper into food. The risk of release increases with longer cooking and preparation time, higher temperatures and the presence of acids such as vinegar or lemon.

Even some commercial trace element supplements contain unnecessarily high amounts of copper in relation to the other constituent elements (especially zinc). Prolonged intake of these products can lead to unfavorable effects pertaining to copper and zinc function (zinc works antagonistically to copper in many places). This is risky if higher doses of the preparations are taken under the impression that more is better.

Wilson's disease is a genetic disorder in which the copper transport protein ceruloplasmin is missing. This results in an increased amount of copper being deposited into tissue. Damage occurs particularly to the brain, liver and kidneys. Externally visible copper deposits in the eyes are typical. Due to brain damage, patients become mentally unstable, irritable, and aggressive and eventually suffer from dementia. Parkinson-like symptoms and other neurological problems also develop.

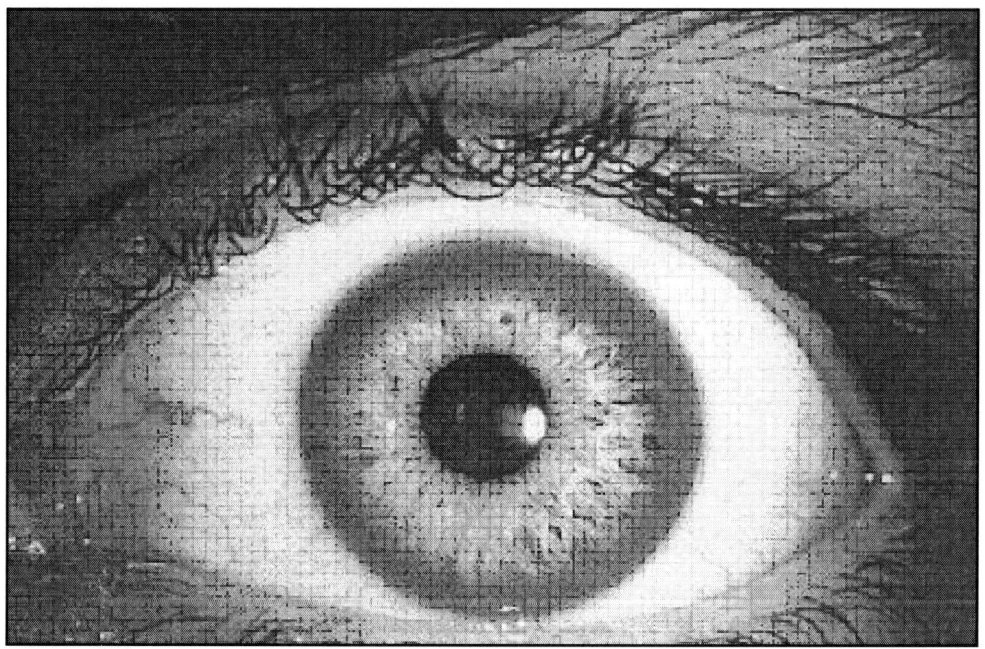

Kayser-Fleischer corneal ring confirms excessive copper deposition in patients with Wilson's disease

Migraine patients can experience a worsening of headaches in response to high copper intake. Estrogens from oral contraceptives can elevate copper levels in women.

Elevated copper levels have also been identified as a factor in post-partum depression, premenstrual tension, psychosis and paranoia (copper acts as a brain stimulant). High copper levels continue to be reported in connection with smoking. Due to the biological antagonism between copper and zinc, elevated copper levels can also arise from zinc-deficient diets. The stimulatory effects of high copper levels on the brain may be reversed by zinc administration and metallothionein support. Copper elimination can be difficult in some cases when the concentration of the copper carrier protein ceruloplasmin is low.

Elevated copper levels have been associated with ADHD (Attention Deficit Hyperactivity Disorder). These individuals experience restlessness, diminished concentration, difficulty sustaining attention, impulsive behavior and academic problems.

In the brain, copper is found largely as a component of monoamine oxidase. Inhibitors of the MAO-A enzyme are used to treat anxiety and depression while inhibitors of the MAO-B enzyme are used to treat Parkinson's disease.

Some researchers have reported a gradual increase in copper levels among the elderly and are considering whether this plays a role in some of the problems associated with aging.

Interesting observations have been made about the behavior of copper in rheumatism. In chronic polyarthritis, copper levels are particularly low in the periosteum. Within the bone, copper levels are reduced to about one half of the normal amount. Decreased bone mineral levels have also been observed (especially calcium, magnesium, iron and zinc).

Copper has anti-inflammatory effects in rheumatism, especially in acute cases. However, copper deficiencies are very difficult to identify using blood tests. Copper is released from deposits (especially from the liver) in response to infection and inflammation. This can lead to an elevation of blood serum and hair mineral measures even in cases where copper is deficient in body tissues.

Occasionally copper deficiencies appear in children, especially if they were raised exclusively on cow's milk, or as a result of prolonged diarrhea.

Copper therapy was popular in antiquity. The ancient Egyptians knew about the importance of copper and its use continued among the ancient Greeks, Romans and Arabs. It was applied internally and externally to treat infections and mental illness. The medieval physician Paracelsus was famous for copper therapies.

Inhalation of copper dust, which is quite rare, leads to a feverish illness after several hours. This is identified by a very high fever with shivers, cough, and joint and muscle pain. Prolonged intake of copper dust leads to a green pigmentation of skin, hair, teeth and gums, as well as inflammation of mucous membranes of the eye and nose. Intake of copper salts in large amounts (such as copper vitriol) leads to the cauterization of stomach and intestinal areas accompanied by vomiting, diarrhea and colic. If this is not fatal, permanent liver and kidney damage often remain.

Copper was the first metal used in the Bronze Age after its melting property was discovered around the fifth and sixth centuries BC. Copper was customarily melted with arsenic. As we know today, this leads to paralysis from chronic arsenic poisoning. Limping has been identified as a characteristic occupational illness among the blacksmiths of this period.

Menkes disease is a rare recessive X-linked illness involving aberrant copper metabolism. It involves external changes to hair (kinky hair), degeneration of the brain, cramping, and osteoporosis, and generally leads to death between the ages of 3 months to 3 years. In a few patients, early intravenous copper administration allows some normal development to proceed.

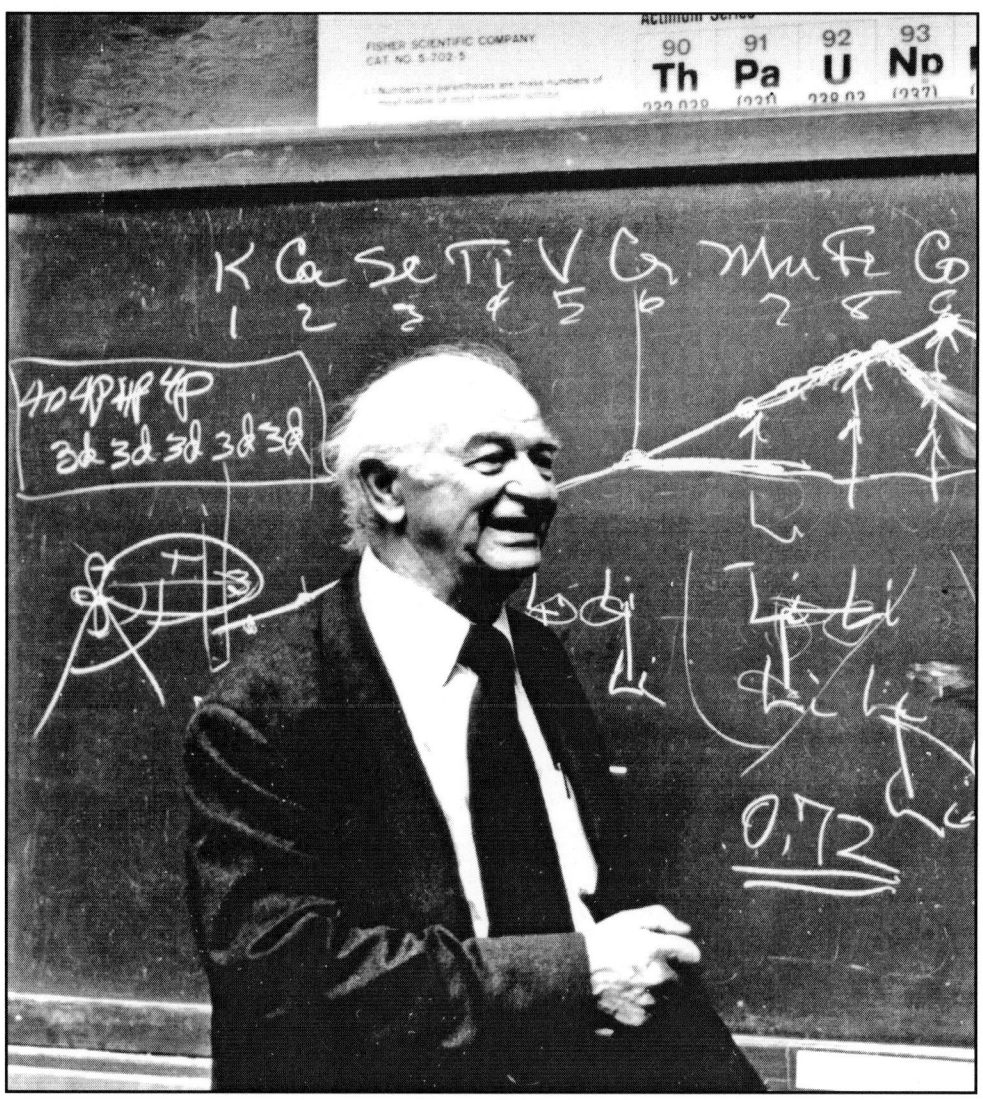

Linus Pauling (1901-1994), Nobel laureate, lecturing at Oregon State University in 1983 on the chemical nature of minerals and metals. Pauling understood well the central biochemical role of minerals having published many papers on mineral and crystal structures. In later years, his main interest was in vitamin C biochemical research. He suggested that people aim for an optimal intake of all micronutrients, including minerals, and made some specific recommendations in his book "How To Live Longer and Feel Better", in which he also emphasized the role of biochemical individuality. He considered micronutrients an important adjunct to standard medical practice. [Picture courtesy of Ava Helen and Linus Pauling Papers, Oregon State University.]

FLUORINE

chemical symbol **F**

Daily requirement: ~2-4 mg (children 0.1-2.5 mg)

Biological significance: debated

Therapeutic applications: controversial application in:
- tooth decay (caries) prevention
- osteoporosis

Negative biological effects: practically only possible through synthetic intake or by fluoride consumed water

Sources: meat, fish
milk
wheat products

FLUORINE

The element that is more poisonous than beneficial

Fluorine is a somewhat problematic element; it has not been conclusively evaluated by medical research yet it has gained a critical use therapeutically.

It is used at a dosage of about 1 mg per day as a treatment against caries in children. However, some researchers believe that adequate fluorine can generally be obtained from the diet (such as the amount required for the hardening of enamel). Sufficient intake of calcium and vitamin D and avoidance of excess sugar is more important for healthy teeth than fluoride treatment.

In certain areas, fluorine is added to drinking water at a concentration of 1 mg/L. In principle, only a very small amount of the drinking water prepared this way is actually consumed. The remaining fluorine could possibly pose a threat to the environment.

Whereas the layperson may only hear success stories about caries treatment, several critical viewpoints exist concerning the negative effects of fluorine. New data from China show neurological impairment including ADD/ADHD due to fluorine intake. Further, more than one million people have crippled skeletons because of high fluorine levels in the drinking water. Some researchers find fluorine to be more toxic than lead – especially in children. As an iodine antagonist, fluorine was used as an anti-thyroid medication prior to 1950. Importantly, a slightly under-functioning thyroid gland during pregnancy can result in a lower IQ in the newborn (in addition to the toxic effect of fluorine). Children "optimally treated" with fluorine since birth have been shown to develop dental fluorosis to some degree as adolescents: small spots develop on the surfaces of teeth, which may also appear discolored. In more distinctive cases, enamel also becomes uneven. Some studies did not show a preventive effect of fluoridation on tooth decay. Some researchers find that fluorine may be cancer-promoting.

People who have amalgam fillings in their teeth should avoid the use of fluoride toothpaste, since this can lead to an increased release of mercury from the fillings.

In much higher doses (75-100 mg per day over several years), sodium fluoride has been used to treat osteoporosis in Germany and a few other countries. However, the effectiveness of this treatment method has been doubted since two double-blind studies in the US during 1989 and 1990 indicated an increase in bone fractures with fluoride treatment.

Fluorine is taken up by the intestines and is excreted through the urine. In certain instances, it can also enter the body through inhalation. In rare cases of high uptake, fluorine can eat away at mucous membranes of the digestive tract (accompanied by nausea, vomiting and bloody diarrhea). Because fluorine takes some time to be excreted, damage to other organs may occur in the meantime as various metabolic pathways are disrupted. Sometimes, mineral water can contain significant amounts of fluorine. Levels above 5 mg/L legally require a note of caution in Europe.

Tooth decay: a dietary problem?

The bacteria naturally found in the mouth survive mainly on sugar. As a by-product of their metabolic activities, these bacteria produce acids such as acetic acid. These acids then attack dental enamel. Some strains of bacteria also use sugar to form insoluble compounds (glucans) that cannot be removed by saliva alone. This leads to a steady increase in tartar lining the teeth, especially in mechanically inaccessible areas (cavities and spaces between teeth). The insoluble compounds impair the uptake of minerals from saliva that are required for the hardening of enamel, and hinder the saliva's ability to neutralize acids produced by bacteria. Bacterial activity is encouraged when saliva can no longer penetrate thicker layers of tartar. A white spot forms, and eventually a cavity develops. Tartar and bacterial activity also lead to inflammation of the gums, which encourages the development of periodontitis, a condition in which gums recede to the point where teeth may fall out.

In third world countries, replacing a natural diet with a "modern" diet has increased the incidence of cavities from rare to the level seen in today's western society. Very few people now do not have these dental problems.

The risk of cavities rises according to the sugar content and stickiness of foods. Bacterial acid production increases as more sugar is available. Sucrose particularly promotes glucan formation and tartar production. While fruits can contain up to 12% sugar, they hardly promote cavities because they do not stick to teeth and their acid content stimulates saliva production (except for bananas and dried fruits).

High amounts of saliva protect tooth enamel, as is the case when chewing is increased through the consumption of whole foods and whole grain products. Infants and children are at particular risk for developing cavities due to the high sugar content of many drinks. Once infants are accustomed to sweet drinks, they often don't want anything else!

A lower incidence of tooth decay has been found in areas with high amounts of molybdenum in soils and food, even if fluorine is taken up in low amounts. Eventually, vanadium deficiencies can also favor tooth decay.

IRON

The element that keeps us going

About 4-5 g of iron is found in an adult human body. 20-30% of this is stored in the spleen, liver, intestinal mucosa and bone marrow. It functions primarily in the formation of red blood pigment (hemoglobin, for the transport of oxygen in red blood cells) and red muscle pigment (myoglobin, for the storage of oxygen, especially in active muscle cells).

In addition to iron, the production of hemoglobin requires copper, vitamin C, vitamin B12 and folic acid.

The absorption and excretion of iron is important. Iron is obtained from meat, fish, whole grain products and vegetables (general rule: the darker the source, the more iron it contains). However, iron-rich vegetables do not provide much value if they are consumed with coffee or tea. The tannins in these drinks react with the iron, preventing it from being absorbed by the body. Even though an average diet may provide the required daily 10-15 mg, fluctuations from the 10% absorption rate often occur.

The absorption of iron is decreased by phosphate, phytate (in whole grain products), tannic acid (in coffee, tea, and red wine), antacids, zinc and manganese. 20% of the iron contained in meat is absorbed.

Deficiencies in iron and vitamin B12 are common among vegetarians. The body absorbs less than 5% of iron consumed in vegetarian sources. Vitamin C, gastric acid and calcium promote the absorption of iron.

Iron is lost from the body at a rate of 1 mg/day through stool, dead skin cells and sweat. Women lose more iron during menstruation.

Typical symptoms of iron deficiency are pale skin, fatigue, loss of appetite, nervousness and irritability, increased susceptibility to infection, headache and sensitivity to weather/meteorological changes, brittle hair and nails. Iron deficiency can be caused by internal or external blood loss, a diet which hinders iron absorption, and by stomach or intestinal tract diseases, especially if gastric acid amounts are inadequate.

Pregnant women were often told to "eat for two." However, this commonly leads to unnecessary weight gain, which may cause problems in later pregnancy and at birth. The current recommendations are more straightforward: take iron "for the blood" and calcium to promote healthy bone development. It is not commonly realized that additional zinc is also recommended for pregnant women.

Iron continued on page 47

IRON

Latin: *Ferrum*; chemical symbol **Fe**

known as an essential element since the 17th-18th century

Normal daily requirement:

children and adults 10-15 mg
women need extra: up to 18 mg
intestinal absorption is about 10%
25 mg for women after 6th month of pregnancy

Functions:

component of red pigment in blood and muscles (hemoglobin and myoglobin); therefore important for blood formation, growth and immune defenses

Therapeutic applications:

for the following deficiency symptoms:
- fatigue, anemia
- weight loss
- growth disturbances
- increased susceptibility to infections
- higher rate of premature births

Sources:

meat, fish, whole grain products, legumes, vegetables, nuts, brewer's yeast, and soy

Note:

absorption is enhanced by:
- vitamin C
- gastric acid
- calcium

absorption is compromised by:
- tannic acid (in coffee, tea and red wine),
- phytate (in whole grain products),
- antacids, zinc and manganese

Iron continued from page 45

In general, medical practitioners and laypersons are aware of iron deficiency issues. It is not, however, common knowledge that the incidence of premature births rises according to the severity of iron deficiency. It is estimated that about 20% of all premature births could be avoided by providing better iron supplementation to pregnant women.

Iron levels among breastfed infants are much better than among those who are fed baby formula. The intestinal tract of an infant can absorb up to 50% of the iron found in breast milk, but only up to 20% of the iron found in cow's milk.

As with many other minerals, overdoses can be just as unfavorable as deficiencies. Iron overload (hemochromatosis) can be even more problematic than iron deficiency. Iron can slowly accumulate due to overactive intestinal absorption (often there is a reason for this) over several years or decades. Only at elevated body levels of 20-40 g will the first symptoms appear. Damage occurs to the following:
- Pancreas: with eventual development of diabetes;
- Skin: often brown/gray pigmentation develops ("Bronze-Diabetes");
- Liver: leading to cirrhosis;
- Heart: disruptions in cardiac rhythm; heart failure;
- Joints: leading to increasing complaints;
- Testes: can lead to impotency or infertility.

Elevated iron intake can occur as a result of high iron content in drinking water, iron cookware or through repetitive blood transfusions. While iron deficiency can be easily identified by laboratory tests even before significant symptoms arise, an investigation of hemochromatosis requires special blood tests to assess the status of the iron transport protein transferrin and the iron storage protein ferritin.

GERMANIUM

chemical symbol **Ge**

Normal daily requirement:
uncertain, ~ 1-3 mg?
not generally regarded as an essential element
therapeutic dosage often 40-60 mg

Functions:
not known

Therapeutic applications*:
due to its immuno-stimulatory
and pain-relieving effects in:
- cancer, leukemia, chemotherapy
- consumptive diseases (diseases leading to consumption of tissue, loss of weight or physical power – tuberculosis, AIDS, cancer, etc.)
- severe pain, especially associated with cancer and severe polyarthritis
- heavy metal intoxication, especially lead, cadmium and mercury

Negative biological effects:
serious kidney damage upon consumption
(has been reported)

Sources:
garlic, ginseng
comfrey
mussels, oysters, tuna
mushrooms
wild rice
spring water from particular areas

*according to advocates

GERMANIUM
The controversial trace element

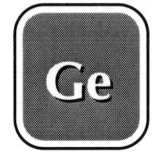

The small group of advocates/supporters and users of germanium are looked at with skepticism and caution. Therefore, few medical practitioners have experience using germanium. Although inorganic germanium compounds were applied in the past, present suggestions focus on organically bound germanium. Since the 1950's, the use of germanium to treat illnesses has been influenced by Dr. K. Asai of Japan, after germanium was discovered in ginseng and Lourdes water.

Organic germanium is taken up quickly by the small intestine (within 3 hours following ingestion) and distributed throughout the entire body. After 12 hours, the majority of the absorbed germanium is excreted unchanged via the kidney.

Patients in Japan were treated with daily dosages of up to 1 g without any significant reports of side effects. In Europe however, some cases of kidney damage were observed. In 1993, Polish pharmacologist and toxicologist Prof. L. Samochowiec conducted a study on animals and human volunteers. Healthy people were given 45 mg of germanium daily for 60 weeks without any evidence of kidney damage.

Those who support the use of germanium report several beneficial effects:
- strengthening of immune defenses, even when the immune system is suppressed, as is often in cancer;
- effective pain relief, especially among cancer and severe polyarthritis patients;
- favorable influence on calcium metabolism and pain relief in osteoporosis;
- improvements in oxygen usage, energy stores, general performance and well-being.

Apparently, germanium has positive effects in different forms of oxygen deficiency, including Raynaud's disease and stroke. A warm or prickling sensation has often been reported when taking germanium at therapeutic doses.

Fungal and microbial infections such as Candida have been observed to respond positively. Germanium is said to release toxic heavy metals such as lead, cadmium and mercury enabling more expedient excretion.

MERCURY

Latin: *Hydrargyrum*; chemical symbol **Hg**

poisonous ☠

Functions: none

Therapeutic applications: none (or only in dental amalgams)

Negative biological effects: acts on liver, kidneys, spleen and
especially brain:
- rapid fatigue, depression
- nervousness, irritability
- decreased memory
- headaches, migraines, nausea
- general decline in well-being
- weight loss
- increased susceptibility to allergic reactions
- stomach aches

Note: sudden onset of other complaints is possible,
especially coinciding with infections and
other zinc deficiency-related symptoms

Sources: dental amalgam
thermometers
fluorescent light bulbs
exposed fish, animals and plants
thimerosal in vaccines and flu shots

MERCURY
That poisonous metal in your dental fillings

Mercury is one of the elements whose toxicity has been known for a long time. While it has only been released in nature in small amounts from decay and volcanic activity, its use has increased significantly within the last century (which consequently increases its release into the environment). Mercury is used in the chlorine, potash and electrical industries, in the manufacturing of batteries, and formerly in railways to produce direct current for their electric systems. It is used industrially in metal manufacturing (including applications in dentistry), in the production of paints, mercury vapor lamps and thermometers, and as an organic compound in disinfectants, preservatives and stains. Mercury was previously used in the medical field to treat syphilis and skin disorders.

In Germany, it is estimated that 280 tonnes of mercury is released into the environment every year due to industrial output. This does not include an additional 60 tonnes released as a result of burning fossil fuels. Burning garbage sets free most of the mercury it contains. A specific type of pollution is developing in the upper layers of soil, where mercury is incorporated into insoluble compounds. The worldwide expansion and scope of environmental pollution caused by mercury is exemplified by the fact that the mercury content in the upper layers of Greenland's glaciers doubled between 1950 and 1980. A similar observation has been made in the feathers of birds kept in captivity. Up until 1940, constant mercury levels of 2 µg/g were found, but in the following years an increase of up to 13 times this amount was recorded. This could be traced back to the use of seed preparation agents that contained mercury. Upon banning these agents, feather mercury levels returned to those found before 1940.

Careless handling of pesticides and chemical treatment agents containing mercury led to mass poisoning in several developing countries. For example, poisonings caused 500 deaths in Iran in 1972. In 1969, Canada temporarily banned the hunting of wild birds due to the burden they were already experiencing from mercury poisoning. However, mercury exposure did not only have an impact on birds. Mercury preparations could also be found on seeds in pig food, which led to poisoning among humans upon consumption of pork. Consequently, the US banned the use of mercury compounds as seed staining agents in 1971.

In Japan, government guidelines suggest that whales and dolphins (who are at the end of the food-chain) should have no more than 0.4 µg/g of mercury in their livers. However, the *New Scientist* (June 2001) reported that the average amount is 370 µg/g, 900 times the allowed limit.

Perhaps the most dramatic example of mercury damage is an obscure appearance of illness in Japan's Minamata Bay. Between 1953 and 1960, over 100 people developed "Minamata disease." This illness was predominantly marked by restlessness and anxiety, followed by serious damage to the nervous system involving cramps and paralysis. There were 48 deaths, and 10% of 400 births developed brain damage. Survivors were left mentally impaired and many experienced symptoms of paralysis. Several years later it was discovered that large volumes of factory waste water containing mercury had been diverted into the bay. Mercury accumulated in fish by passing through the food chain, eventually reaching humans. Fish usually contain high levels of selenium, which has a protective effect against mercury (explained in the Selenium chapter). High selenium levels allow people who consume a lot of fish (like the Japanese) to better deal with mercury contamination.

Metallic mercury normally passes through the intestinal tract and is excreted unchanged. However, small amounts can become trapped between intestinal folds and may be absorbed over longer periods of time. On the other hand, mercury released by broken thermometers or mercury lamps is much more dangerous. Mercury particles can quickly disappear into floor crevices and turn into vapor over time, presenting a prolonged contamination risk.

Mercury poisoning can be acute, sub-acute or chronic depending on the dosage and duration of exposure. Chronic mercury poisoning causes head and neck pain, trembling, loss of teeth (with a mercury lining on the gums), diarrhea, kidney and nerve damage as well as sensory, speech, auditory, vision, memory and locomotive disturbances up to and including hallucinations.

Intake of larger amounts within a short period of time such as with the inhalation of mercury vapors or the swallowing of mercury compounds causes acute poisoning. Localized inflammation occurs at the point of contact. At this point vomiting may occur, which may in fact save the victim's life. Kidney damage is often the result, with a fatal outcome if allowed to progress to complete kidney failure.

Occupational mercury poisoning is covered by worker's compensation and insured through wage indemnity programs.

Liver, kidneys, spleen and brain are primary locations for mercury deposition within the body.

The excretion of mercury is very slow. However, it can be enhanced by a selenium-rich diet, sulfur-containing amino acids, zinc and vitamins B1, B6, A, C, and E.

Serious mercury poisoning is treated with drugs (especially DMPA/DMPS and DMSA) that bind mercury to form complexes for elimination. This requires medical supervision since these chelating agents (agents that grab metal ions) also bind to other metals in the same periodic row such as copper and zinc. In the periodic table of elements, mercury is found exactly 2 rows under zinc and 1 row under cadmium.

The results of a 1990/1992 environmental government survey on mercury in Germany described appropriate indicators for mercury poisoning. While inorganic mercury levels are reflected by urinanalysis, blood tests are better able to demonstrate organic mercury poisoning. The latter generally causes a higher toxicity and is also suited to hair mineral analysis. Average mercury levels were found to be 0.5 µg/L in urine and 0.3 µg/L in blood in the general population.

Problems associated with amalgam fillings

An amalgam is a combination of mercury, silver, copper and tin (and sometimes other metals). Favored for its excellent malleability and low cost, amalgams have been used in dental fillings for decades. All other materials, including tooth replacement, are significantly more expensive. Gold fillings can also cause undesirable effects in some cases due to the use of other metals contained. Fillings should be free of palladium and have a gold content of at least 90%.

Various amalgams are available; for example, one type contains selenium. On average, amalgams contain about 40% mercury. Such a filling in the tooth leads to prolonged mercury exposure. This occurs due to slow electrolytic decomposition, chemical reactions, mechanical abrasion and vaporization at a minute but cumulative level. The risk for mercury-elevation is greater in children than in adults. The release of mercury from fillings is promoted by acidic foods and drinks (depending on their strength and length of time in contact with teeth), fluoride toothpaste, other metals inside the mouth, and by intensive chewing. Some studies show a decrease in immunoglobulins in blood several minutes after chewing gum due to the release of mercury.

Since hair mineral analysis generally reflects recent mercury levels but does not indicate mercury deposition within inner organs, there is a specialized diagnostic tool known as the mercury mobilization test. DMPS, a chelating agent also used in the treatment of mercury poisoning, is administered intravenously at a dosage of 3 mg/kg body weight. Since it has an absorption rate of about 1/3, it can also be given as a 100-200 mg capsule on an empty stomach. Urine mercury levels are measured before and after taking DMPS. In principle, this process also causes other heavy metals and trace elements to be excreted in the following order: zinc, copper, arsenic, mercury, lead, iron, cadmium, nickel, and then chromium.

High levels of copper, lead and cadmium can reduce the excretion of mercury to such an extent that repetitive mobilization tests have to be performed in order for mercury to become sufficiently measurable in the urine. Zinc must be supplemented when performing repeated mobilizations due to its high rate of excretion. Zinc deficiency is not uncommon and will enhance the negative biological effects of mercury. Conversely, slightly elevated mercury levels can be reversed through prolonged zinc and selenium intake. All work involving amalgam fillings (including their removal) poses a special risk of mercury exposure. Specific recommendations protect dentists and patients involved in these procedures.

Children, pregnant women or anyone with organ damage (especially problems with the nervous system) should be considered highly sensitive to mercury and other heavy metals.

Children should definitely not receive amalgam fillings, mainly because their primary teeth are eventually replaced. Dentists should continue to stress regular dental hygiene as a preventive measure.

The following consequences of amalgam fillings have been reported:
- premature fatigue, depression;
- irritability, anxiety;
- diminished memory;
- headaches and migraines, nausea, vision disturbances;
- decrease in general well-being, including weight loss;
- stomach ache;
- increased susceptibility to allergies.

The biological half-life of mercury is not the same in every organ: in the blood, the half-life is three months; versus the brain where the half-life is about 18 years (six months with therapeutic mobilization). It should be noted that blood analysis only determines acute toxicity or poisoning.

Mercury toxicity can exist for several years without noticeable symptoms, but acute health problems can appear suddenly. For example, on the occasion of an infection (which leads to an increased requirement for zinc), mercury ions can accumulate, tax the immune system, and result in the quicker onset of symptoms. Other situations which place a demand on the body's zinc or selenium stores can induce similar effects. Suppressed zinc levels can also lead to increased copper levels due to zinc-copper antagonism.

Some medical practitioners and dentists regard dental amalgams as poisonous. Ironically, the first dentists/physicians who brought mercury dental amalgams/fillings to America were arrested as charlatans. Dental amalgams exert a dangerous influence on the internal body even though they are placed in the tooth.

Thimerosal-containing vaccines administered before 6 months of age are associated with developmental disorders including speech/language disorders, and ADHD. Thimerosal is a preservative that contains ethyl mercury. Recently, European and American regulatory authorities recommended the phasing out of thimerosal. An entirely new thimerosal-free childhood vaccine product line is now on the market. Thimerosal preservatives are also found in flu shots and other drugs. The body depends on the metallothionein series of proteins to bind and eliminate mercury. A select portion of the population has compromised metallothionein function. The Pfeiffer Centre in Chicago has often found compromised metallothionein function in autistic patients.

Environmental disasters involving mercury exposure are handled with special decontamination procedures. Similarly there are special decontamination procedures for disposing of extracted teeth which have dental amalgams. In Europe, the concentration of airborne mercury allowed in a room in a house is 1/400th of that in a person's mouth. In Europe drinking water is allowed to contain a maximum of 1 µg/L (or 0.001 mg/L) of mercury but approximately 700 µg/L (0.7 mg/L) is released from a dental amalgam when you chew gum. If the body's water stores contained 700 µg/L of mercury, this would exceed the limits of safe drinking water.

In many tropical countries, gold (one quarter of the world's production) is produced in primitive but effective ways by mercury-extraction. Gold-containing matter is mixed with mercury, which acts as a dissolving agent, and later the mercury is removed by evaporation (the by-products of which pollute even distant regions). In these mining areas, many people suffer from mercury poisoning. Investigators found people with high mercury values but no (or not yet apparent) symptoms, and other people with typical symptoms but normal values. This interesting observation raises a question: is there a "normal" level of poison for a sensitive person? Due to biochemical individuality, one does not know how sensitive an individual will be to a poison.

The standard fish staple of the American diet, canned tuna fish, has been involved in a constant battle in California to prevent it from being banned from supermarkets because of its mercury levels. However, far more insidious than mercury contamination are the increasing levels of PCBs (polychlorinated biphenyls) and dioxins in fish. Although the production of PCBs was stopped in 1977, it will take decades to break down PCBs and dioxins. Today, the blood levels of Vietnamese residents still contain marked levels of dioxin from agent orange exposure.

IODINE

chemical symbol **I**

recognized as an essential element in 1950

Normal daily requirement:
140 µg (ages 1-9)
200 µg (after the age of 9)
250 µg (pregnant women)

Functions:
component of thyroid hormone

Therapeutic applications:
used to treat the following
deficiency symptoms:
- enlargement of the thyroid gland (goiter)
- fatigue
- diminished concentration
- reduced growth and slow
  mental development in children

Sources:
sea salt, iodized table salt
shelled seafood and ocean fish
apples, fruit, spinach

Note:
beets and cabbage can contain antagonists

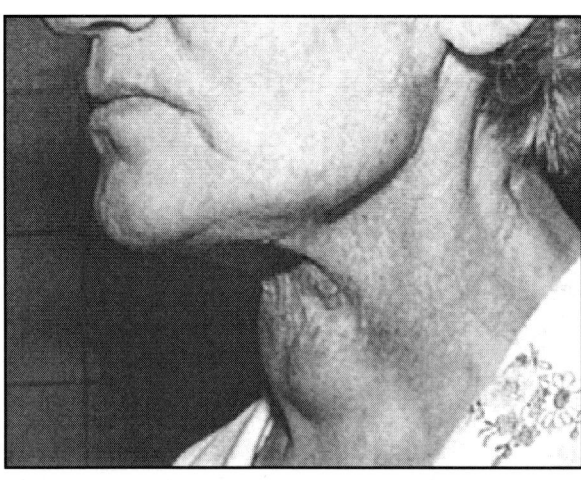 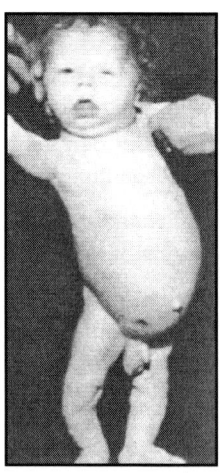

IODINE DEFICIENCY: *left: enlargement of the thyroid gland (goiter) right: an infant with myxedema due to iodine deficiency*

IODINE

The element contained in thyroid hormone

An adult human body contains about 10-30 mg of iodine (primarily in the thyroid gland). As a component of the thyroid hormones thyroxine and triiodothyronine (also known as T4 and T3), iodine is essential to human life. These hormones are responsible for the rate of energy metabolism and they are also important for growth and mental development in children. An under-active thyroid will cause metabolic functions to slow down, leaving a person tired, depressed, and sensitive to cold with decreased drive and an increased need to sleep.

Iodine deficiency leads to enlargement of the thyroid gland in 1-6% of newborns. This contributes to a delay in bone maturation and brain development (they appear quiet and passive). If this is promptly recognized and treated, growth and mental development can be normalized. A 1994 study in Germany identified iodine deficiency and goiter formation among 60% of women whose average daily iodine intake was under 100 µg (the minimum requirement recommended by the WHO).

About 12 billion people worldwide live in iodine-deficient areas. In China, millions of people are mentally handicapped due to iodine deficiency. Some villages exist in which over half of the population is handicapped, requiring many families to rely on outside help to manage their farms. For this reason, a campaign was started in India in 1986 to make the addition of iodine to table salt mandatory by law. This drastically reduced the frequency of mentally handicapped newborns from 9.8% to 1.4%. In India, the yearly transport of 2.3 million tonnes of salt is regarded with as high a priority as military transport.

The iodine content of food and drinking water is dependent on the iodine content of soil. In particular areas where the upper soil layers were washed out during the Ice Age ("end moraine areas") contain little iodine in their soils or ground water. This applies especially to the Alp region (central Europe, Austria, Switzerland). Areas closer to the ocean become richer in iodine. Due to their high consumption of seafood, people who live on islands or in coastal regions rarely suffer from iodine deficiency.

Iodine is obtained primarily from ocean fish, sea salt/iodized salt, and from certain vegetables (depending on soil iodine content). It is almost completely taken up by the small intestine. Cabbage, beets and soy products contain natural compounds (goitrogens) that inhibit the uptake of iodine in the thyroid. These should therefore be avoided by anyone with a thyroid condition. Iodine deficiency can be worsened by the following: high amounts of chloride (from table salt hidden in many foods) or by other halogens such as fluorine and bromine; lithium treatment; and perhaps by excess cobalt intake.

The body tries to compensate for iodine deficiency by increasing thyroid gland production through growth, but this does not always succeed. Hypothyroid conditions should be treated promptly, otherwise knots, cysts, calcifications or, in rare cases, thyroid cancer may occur.

In medicine, iodine is used in tinctures and solutions to treat wounds because of its antiseptic and bactericidal actions. It is also used to increase contrast in x-rays, and, in its radioactive form, it is applied as a diagnostic tool to assess thyroid iodine uptake (increased in hyperthyroidism).

Overdose symptoms in Graves' disease (Basedow-type overactive thyroid) and iodine-induced acne usually only appear as a result of very high doses – around five times the recommended daily dosage. Most often, these are isolated occurrences affecting highly sensitive patients. Normally, an overactive thyroid is associated with other diseases. Allergic reactions from x-ray contrasting agents or disinfectants containing iodine are more common.

In Germany, one in seven people is affected by iodine deficiency. The incidence is eight times higher in Bavaria compared to northern Germany. This makes Germany the country with the highest incidence of iodine deficiency and goiter in Europe. The WHO estimates that 400 billion people worldwide are affected. For decades, iodized salt has been the only available salt in Switzerland. Conversely, in the former West German region, iodine was treated almost as if it was a dangerous substance. Iodized salt has only been regulated and approved for use in the food industry there since 1990. If Switzerland's 90% decline in thyroid disease and the resultant savings to health care costs could be transferred to the former West Germany, an estimated half billion euro (equivalent to approximately half billion USD) could be saved per annum. The use of iodized salt in former East Germany led to results similar to those observed in Switzerland. Inclusion of the bad "West German" salt supply had far reaching effects after re-unification of East and West Germany in 1989. The health progress of "East Germany" was eradicated within 5 years (1994 data).

The strict regulation of iodized salt in Germany is due to unwarranted bureaucratic restriction. Other chemicals and artificial colors and flavors can pose a greater risk to the public but are permitted for use in the food industry. In principle, regular table salt could be used in a suicide attempt; that is, if a person could resolve to take 30 g of salt all at once (the equivalent lethal dose for an adult). An average adult only requires 3-5 g (RDA) of iodized table salt per day.

Iodine deficiency can also arise as a result of restrictive diets. For example, a diet free of eggs or cow's milk is sometimes recommended for children with chronic skin conditions such as eczema and neurodermatitis. Such a "hypoallergenic" diet is very low in iodine.

Radioactive iodine-131 resulting from nuclear reactor accidents accumulates in the thyroid and has been associated with thyroid cancer. A healthy thyroid will only absorb 10-20% of the partly radioactive iodine found in food. In iodine deficiency, this uptake rises to 90%! After the Chernobyl nuclear accident, iodine tablets were available in German pharmacies at higher dosages (at doses previously used for the prevention of goiter). The intention was to saturate the thyroid with iodine as quickly as possible to decrease the uptake of radioactive iodine for a period of time. Since iodine deficiency is not rare in Germany, it should be taken into consideration that the thyroid is very sensitive to these unaccustomed iodine dosages. In some cases where goiter is present, a single dose of 0.5-1 mg can disrupt the thyroid and bring about sudden over-activity. Instead of the 0.1 mg usually found in goiter treatment medications, some of the tablets given out in response to the accident contained up to 100 mg of iodine.

Radioactive iodine can cause genetic changes in reproductive glands. It can also contribute to growth disturbances in children.

Since 1991, the following thyroid hormone link has been confirmed in humans (previously, this was known only in animals). Tetraiodothyroxine (also known as thyroxine or T4) is converted into the more biologically active form triiodothyronine (T3) by a type-I-5' deiodase enzyme. This enzyme is found to have the trace element selenium in its active center. Therefore, not only iodine deficiency, but also selenium deficiency can lead to under-active thyroid function! Peroxides formed in the thyroid via thyroperoxidase deactivate the selenium-dependent glutathione peroxidase.

The conversion of T4 to the much more biologically active T3 is reduced in iron-deficient states and may contribute to the symptoms of iron-deficiency.

Reliable iodine values can be measured with hair mineral analysis when the ICP technique is combined with mass spectrography (see Section 2).

POTASSIUM

chemical symbol **K**

Normal daily requirement: adults 3-4 g; infants 0.3 g
- therapeutic dosage for children dependent on age and weight
- doses above the normal daily requirement only under medical supervision

Functions: potassium is important for:
- conduction of impulses in nerve and muscle cells including heart muscle cells
- kidney function
- water and acid/base regulation

Therapeutic applications: disturbances in cardiac rhythm
constipation, diarrhea/vomiting, edema
muscle weakness, poor circulation
high blood pressure
potassium loss due to physical activity

Negative biological effects: cardiac arrhythmias caused by excess potassium are only possible as a result of medications or potassium injections

Sources: fruit (especially bananas)
vegetables, potatoes
milk, cheese, meat, nuts

Potassium deficiency: can be caused by increased potassium loss, inadequate potassium intake, and by a variety of medications. These include some drugs used to treat high blood pressure, diuretics, and above all, laxatives. Regular, prolonged use of laxatives creates a vicious cycle of problems. Laxatives cause the body to lose potassium via the elimination of bowel waste products. Potassium deficiency, in turn, decreases intestinal motility, which is made worse by taking more laxative.

Cortisone preparations also lead to potassium deficiency. Anorexia, crash diets, prolonged mineral loss due to vomiting, diarrhea or wound secretion (particularly relevant in large surface area burns) are all risk factors for potassium deficiency.

POTASSIUM

The muscle performance element

Potassium is the most abundant element in the human body after calcium and phosphorous. Of the 140 g found in an adult human body, 98% is found within cells (intracellular) and only 2% is extracellular. The opposite is true for sodium. These concentration differences are important for the formation and conduction of electrical impulses in muscle cells and nerves.

Potassium is also important for water and acid/base regulation. It acts as an activator of numerous enzymes, especially those involved in the metabolism of sugar.

Potassium deficiency leads to muscle weakness and contributes to muscle cramps. This is especially relevant to athletes since they lose a lot of potassium (as well as magnesium and zinc) through perspiration. Muscle performance can drop considerably; cramping may even cause an athlete to pull out of competition. Various mineral drinks target athletes by promising better performance. Recreational athletes can mix equal parts of fruit juice and water to make a sports drink that is almost as effective, tastes better and is more economical.

Adults normally require 3-4 g of potassium daily. Up to 10 g can be required during periods of intense physical activity due to mineral loss as a result of perspiration. Potassium deficiency is not immediately noticeable as a decrease in well-being, therefore even experienced athletes can be deceived and may continue training until their performance drops sharply. Some instances have occurred in which athletes were not able to identify their prolonged performance lows as a potassium deficiency in time for competition. Following potassium intake, muscles usually require some time to recover and return to their previous level of performance. Prolonged potassium deficiency leads to disruptions in cardiac function (especially cardiac rhythm disturbances), decreases in blood pressure and circulation, constipation and disturbance of kidney function.

Potassium is primarily excreted by the kidneys (90%). The other 10% is excreted in the stool. Consequently, disturbances to potassium regulation often occur as a result of kidney disease or diuretic use. Some potassium-sparing diuretics can sometimes even cause hyperkalemia when coadministered with potassium or ACE inhibitors, or when renal function is compromised.

LITHIUM

chemical symbol **Li**

probably essential in very small amounts

Daily requirement: unknown (~1-2 mg?)

Functions: unknown

Therapeutic applications: recurring depression and mania (dosage dependent on blood values)

Horton's neuralgia, migraines

weakened immunity, especially when leukocytes are diminished

cancer therapy, 30-60 mg/day

Negative biological effects: overdosage (determined by blood analysis) leads to trembling of hands followed by nausea and diarrhea, then disturbances of heart and brain

Sources: almost all foods contain trace amounts of lithium
- in water, lithium content correlates with the amount of calcification (some mineral waters have higher amounts of lithium)
- relatively high lithium content in tobacco

LITHIUM

Poisonous in some cases, beneficial in others

As the third element of the periodic table, lithium is the lightest metal. Lithium compounds are often used in industrial applications such as batteries.

Even though lithium-dependent physiological and biochemical functions have not yet been identified, lithium does seem to antagonize the effects of potassium, calcium and magnesium. Some enzymes that are activated by potassium are inhibited by lithium. There is also a competitive relationship with sodium in the renal tubule: lithium and sodium compete for reabsorption.

Within the body, lithium is most abundant in the lymph nodes (0.2 ppm), followed by the brain and bone marrow. 95% of the amount contained in the diet is taken up in the blood. 0.1-3 mg is taken up from the diet every day. Excretion occurs almost exclusively through the urine. Only small amounts are excreted through perspiration and by the intestinal tract.

US studies have identified an increased incidence of psychiatric disorders, mental instability, drug abuse and cardiac disease in lithium-poor regions. Perhaps the relatively high lithium content in tobacco contributes to the calming effect experienced by many smokers.

Various healing sources used by the ancient Romans to treat depression have now been found to have lithium content. In the 19th century, lithium salts were used to treat kidney stones. In 1949, a physician in Australia identified lithium as the beneficial factor in the drinking water of one fountain after it was observed that it led to improvements in mental well-being among several people. Since then, the use of lithium to treat recurring depression and mania has increased. Under medical supervision, especially when blood values are monitored, toxic side effects associated with high dosages rarely occur. The overdose symptom of diarrhea usually diminishes lithium uptake thereby counteracting overdose. At the beginning of lithium treatment, side effects such as diarrhea, increased water excretion and trembling can occur. These side effects may disappear during the course of treatment.

Caution must be exercised due to the narrow therapeutic range of lithium. This presents two possible problems. On one hand, insufficient dosage may not yield a therapeutic response while on the other hand, if the dosage is too high, a toxic buildup may occur. Serum concentrations of 0.6-0.8 (up to 1.0) mmol/L are optimal for treatment. The first overdose symptoms usually occur at 1.2 mmol/L and poisoning symptoms appear at 1.6-2.0 mmol/L. An insufficient dose, which does not cause any complaints, would only be noticed upon recurrence of depression or mania (especially if regular blood tests are not carried out). The toxic effect of lithium can be decreased by potassium and calcium intake without impairing lithium's therapeutic effects.

At higher doses, iodine regulation in the thyroid gland can be influenced. Long-term lithium treatment leads to diminished T3 and T4 and an enlarged thyroid in 5% of patients. In hyperthyroidism, when the thyroid is often enlarged, the goal is to decrease T3 and T4 levels. For this purpose, you can take lithium, especially in treating thyrotoxicosis (hyperthyroidism) and therapy-resistant iodine-induced thyroid hyperactivity.

One particular aspect sometimes causes difficulties when measuring lithium blood values. Similar to potassium, lithium is found primarily within cells; therefore, it is more abundant inside red blood cells than in the blood plasma used for the analysis. Incorrect blood sampling techniques can lead to the rupture of red blood cells (hemolysis), allowing intracellular lithium to raise the plasma reading. If the lithium dosage is lowered based on this reading, recurrence of illness could develop. This is also an example of the difficulty and error possible in diagnostic lab analyses.

Other positive effects of lithium include:
- relief of migraines following relatively low oral doses of lithium (no lab analyses required).
- occasional alleviation of Horton's neuralgia (a form of migraine affecting men in particular) when unresponsive to other treatment approaches.
- improved vitamin B12 and folic acid uptake and a general increase in physical performance.
- a supportive effect against inflammation (including rheumatism) and fungal infections.
- beneficial in ointments to treat herpes infections, psoriasis and sebaceous eczema.

The use of lithium as an immune stimulant and in cancer therapy has recently increased (30-60 mg/day equivalent to 150-300 mg lithium carbonate; reduced dosage if kidney function is compromised). It has been observed to reduce white blood cell loss and bone marrow damage resulting from cancer chemotherapy and cancer radiation therapy. Lithium's role in the management of the conditions mentioned above is probably based on its ability to intervene with arachidonic acid pathways that hinder prostaglandin PGE-1 synthesis.

Lithium in nerve cell physiology

In neurons, lithium restores the electrical membrane by removing excess sodium from within the cell. Rat studies suggest that lithium attaches to glutamate receptors and decreases calcium influx and glutamate toxicity thus preventing nerve cell hyperactivity and calcium overload. Lithium thus has a neuroprotective effect by reducing glutamate induced cytotoxicity (which causes nerve degeneration) and also has an anti-anxiety effect by calming overstimulated nerve cells. High doses of lithium can lower dopamine release while low doses can stimulate serotonin formation. The former may be useful for its anti-anxiety effect while the latter may be useful as an antidepressant.

Various forms of lithium for clinical use

There is some indication that lithium orotate might be effective in much lower doses (and thereby less toxic) than lithium carbonate or lithium citrate. Orotate is a good carrier of minerals and transports them more efficiently into and within cells.

When using lithium orotate, less than 5 mg of elemental lithium may be all that is needed to acheive therapeutic benefit. Lithium carbonate is the most commonly prescribed form of lithium and requires mandatory and frequent blood serum monitoring to avoid toxicity. Since there is no significant increase in blood serum levels when using the low-dose orotate form, blood serum monitoring is not as useful here. Reduced availability of thyroid hormones can cause fatigue (seen also in low-dose lithium orotate therapy). It is therefore useful, regardless of which form of lithium is used, to obtain baseline and follow-up measurements of the peripheral thyroid hormones T3 and T4.

In general, when using lithium salts, practitioners do well to implement regular blood testing to rule out associated problems with kidney function (creatinine clearance), thyroid hormone availability (and thyroid enlargement), dehydration, and potassium and sodium deficiency.

MAGNESIUM

chemical symbol **Mg**

recognized as an essential element in 1931

Normal daily requirement: adults 300-400 mg
during pregnancy/nursing +30%
therapeutic dosage approximately equal to
missing portion of daily requirement

Functions: electrolyte, enzyme activator and
structural component of organic compounds

Therapeutic applications: to treat deficiency symptoms of the CNS:
- headaches, migraines, dizziness, nausea,
  impaired concentration, nervousness,
  anxiety, depression, malaise

circulatory system:
- cramped blood vessels, including heart vessels
- cardiac arrhythmias

muscular system:
- muscle cramps and spasms, especially in calves
- tingling, numbness, tetany

internal organs:
- cramps in sphincters of the stomach,
  bladder and intestines
- cramping of gall ducts, stomach and
  intestinal tract and uterus

Negative biological effects: diarrhea following oral overdose

Sources: whole grain products, especially wheat germ
legumes, vegetables, mushrooms,
brewer's yeast, bananas, raisins

**Magnesium deficiency
is promoted by:** diets low in magnesium: high in sugar and fat
crash diets, alcohol
disturbances in intestinal uptake such as
during intestinal illnesses, diarrhea and
abuse of laxatives, kidney disease and use of
diuretics

MAGNESIUM
The ubiquitous element with numerous clinical applications

The earth's crust consists of 2.5% magnesium. In ocean water, it is the most abundant metal. Magnesium is an indispensable substance for all living organisms. As the central atom of the chlorophyll molecule, it is required by plants to convert the sun's energy into chemically bound energy (photosynthesis). In many respects, magnesium is a general requirement for life on earth.

Although the medical importance of magnesium has been known for many years, it still receives little consideration as a therapeutic element. Magnesium takes part in many essential metabolic pathways, is found in nearly all cells, and activates over 300 enzymes (especially those involved in the metabolism of amino acids, carbohydrates, fats and steroids). Magnesium is also important for the stability and permeability of biological membranes. In many places it is a calcium antagonist.

The adult human body contains about 25-35 g of magnesium. About 50-60% of this is bound in bone, while considerable amounts are found in soft tissue, muscle and the liver. Blood plasma (holding only 0.3% of the body's total magnesium) and fatty tissue contain very little magnesium.

Intestinal absorption of magnesium depends on its availability and the amount required by the organism. About 40-60% of the magnesium found in foods is absorbed. This can fall to 25% or – in cases of magnesium deficiency – can rise to 75%. Intestinal uptake can be hindered by high fat and protein intake, phosphate-rich foods (e.g. soft drinks, soft ice cream), iron (forms insoluble compounds), coffee, alcohol, and preservatives such as oxalic acid and benzoic acid. A diet high in fiber can also lead to diminished magnesium absorption due to an elevated phytate levels.

Conversely, magnesium uptake is enhanced by vitamins B1, B6, C, D, and E. Magnesium is excreted primarily by the kidneys, and also through gastric juices in small amounts. A variable amount is excreted through perspiration. This amount should not be underestimated in athletes.

In principle, any illness in the kidneys and stomach/intestinal tract can lead to magnesium regulation disturbances. By far the most significant factor concerning magnesium deficiency is an inadequate magnesium intake due to "modern" eating habits, including the depletion of magnesium through certain cooking and food washing methods. 18 bananas, 1 kg salmon, 1 kg cheese or 1.4 kg potatoes cover the daily requirement for an adult. The magnesium content in drinking water is also of nutritional value. While soft water often contains about 2.5 mg/L, hard water can contain up to 30 mg/L and thus serves as a good source of magnesium. Besides removing calcium, decalcification systems also take out magnesium. Intensive agricultural approaches use artificial fertilizers, which often do not contain magnesium (but increase corn production), and food processing techniques reduce the magnesium content in our diet.

Some examples of foods high in magnesium are whole grain products, legumes, vegetables, nuts and bananas. Items especially low in magnesium such as baked goods, white bread, pasta, sweets and fats should only be consumed in moderation, particularly if magnesium deficiency exists.

Magnesium overdose (including magnesium from supplement sources) is practically impossible due to continuous intestinal regulation: magnesium is absorbed according to the body's needs. Therefore, magnesium overdose is only possible from magnesium injections or in people with kidney disease (where magnesium excretion is greatly reduced).

Magnesium supplements are advertised in some medical journals along with statements saying: "magnesium deficiency symptoms appear before blood values decline." This suggests a potential problem with magnesium blood testing. Even if blood serum values appear normal, magnesium deficiency may already have developed within the cells and be causing symptoms.

Magnesium is usually measured in the blood serum. The normal range is 0.7-1.0 mmol/L (this value varies somewhat according to the standard of measurement). Lower values are considered a reason for starting magnesium supplementation. In comparison to serum values, the magnesium content of red blood cells is three times higher. Thus, regular laboratory diagnostic methods encounter problems identifying slight magnesium deficiencies. In addition, some experts recommend a diet that is strictly balanced in magnesium, calcium and phosphate over a period of 48 hours in order to establish reliable blood serum values. However, such a diet is hardly feasible for most people. Hair mineral analysis can offer an earlier indication of magnesium deficiency. In some cases (most likely due to an increased mobilization from bone deposits), magnesium values appear above the normal range.

It is not surprising that magnesium deficiency can cause a variety of complaints. Day-to-day changes can easily be misinterpreted as psychosomatic complaints.

Magnesium and the central nervous system

Tension headaches, migraines, dizziness, nausea, nervousness and mood disturbances (including depression) can appear as a result of magnesium deficiency. The body reacts to periods of stress by releasing the "stress hormones" – adrenaline and glucocorticoids. This increases the release of magnesium from cells in exchange for calcium. The elevated amount of magnesium released into the bloodstream is eventually lost through the urine. Long-term stress can lead to intracellular magnesium deficiency creating a vicious cycle in which stress reactions and magnesium deficiency perpetuate. In these cases, magnesium supplementation can decrease the extent of stress hormone release.

Some authors have reported that a magnesium injection (75 mg released very slowly into a vein) can alleviate the start of a migraine attack within 15-30 minutes. This has also been used as a diagnostic red flag for migraine headaches versus other types of headaches that do not respond adequately to magnesium.

An increased incidence of magnesium deficiency has also been reported among patients with temporary cerebral circulation disturbances.

Evening magnesium supplementation has alleviated sleep disturbances among unstable elderly patients. A similar effect has also been reported with evening calcium supplementation.

Magnesium deficiency can cause an under-active autonomic nervous system leading to low blood pressure and poor circulatory system performance among younger people.

Magnesium and the cardiac circulatory system

Magnesium deficiency is often associated with common heart conditions such as heart muscle weakness, angina pectoris and cardiac arrhythmias. In cases where diuretics and digitalis are used for treatment, urinary magnesium excretion increases (also found in patients with secondary hyperaldosteronism). Clinical experience has established the practice of controlling both potassium and magnesium levels during digitalis treatment. Cardiac rhythm disturbances can often be alleviated by magnesium supplementation.

The role of magnesium in cardiac circulatory problems and especially in acute heart attacks is under investigation. A sudden release of magnesium from heart muscle cells occurs during heart attack, which can be prevented by sufficient magnesium concentrations in the bloodstream. In this case, magnesium acts as a natural calcium antagonist. Insufficient magnesium levels cause a shift of calcium from cells to the blood, leading to coronary artery spasms. Some studies have observed a lower incidence of infarction, cardiac arrhythmia and death when magnesium supplementation was included in the treatment.

Magnesium's beneficial effects have also been reported in the treatment of arterial circulatory problems in the arms and legs. Magnesium can also help patients experiencing spasms of retinal blood vessels that lead to a disturbing flickering in the field of vision. Complaints that respond to magnesium supplementation do not require elaborate and comprehensive diagnostic testing to identify the cause of the visual disturbances. These investigations are burdensome for the patient and the health care system. Patients are sometimes referred to psychotherapy if the diagnosis is inconclusive.

The increased constriction of blood vessels in response to magnesium deficiency can encourage high blood pressure in some people. Calcium antagonists are often used to treat high blood pressure. Considering their tolerability and lower cost, magnesium supplements could complement or replace these drugs. This seems especially relevant in high blood pressure cases.

Magnesium stabilizes blood platelets and therefore lowers the risk of platelet aggregation and thrombosis. This can be therapeutically useful following surgical operations.

Magnesium and the muscular system

Calf cramps – often induced by exercise – are typical and common symptoms of magnesium deficiency. The cramps can even be triggered by an evening dance class.

Tetany is a disorder often involving cumulative attacks of anxiety, numbness, painful sensations (on the mouth, tongue, hands and feet), as well as painful muscle cramping (in hands and feet, often causing "paw-like" hand contortions). For some patients, magnesium deficiency is a causative factor and their condition improves in response to magnesium supplementation. These symptoms can also occur due to calcium deficiency.

Magnesium and inner organs

Cramping of the sphincter muscles in the esophageal, stomach, intestinal and bladder regions is a common symptom of magnesium deficiency. Cramping can also develop in the remaining muscles of the stomach, intestine, larynx, bronchi (asthma patients) and in the ducts of the gall bladder and pancreas. Menstrual cramps are often alleviated by magnesium supplementation, which normalizes prostaglandin regulation.

Magnesium and pregnancy

Magnesium deficiency accompanied by calf cramping is relatively common during pregnancy. Many medical practitioners specializing in women's health are aware that magnesium deficiency is associated with a higher incidence of miscarriage and premature birth. Since magnesium helps to relax the muscles of the uterus, it works well in preventing premature contractions.

In the US, magnesium has often been administered as an effective infusion in these situations – even in more serious cases of eclampsia.

Due to their estrogen content, oral contraceptives lower serum magnesium levels by 15-30%. During pregnancy, the body also produces an increased amount of estrogen. In 1988, it was calculated that the cost of providing magnesium supplements for 600,000 women in Germany from their seventh week of pregnancy onward would total 70 million Euro (~70 million USD). Figuring the cost of hospitalization at 150 Euro per day, it was estimated that 135 million Euro would be saved yearly due to shortened hospital stays. In addition, 65 million Euro would be saved by eliminating the intensive care services of the 31,500 infants affected.

Magnesium and kidney disease

The kidneys normally excrete one third of the magnesium absorbed by the body. This process can be disrupted in kidney diseases. When kidney function becomes compromised (when blood creatinine values are over 6 mg/100 ml) magnesium is no longer excreted. If these patients are taking additional vitamin D for bone conditions, the intestinal absorption of magnesium can increase and result in even greater serum magnesium concentrations.

Magnesium loss in addition to protein loss has been observed in some chronic kidney diseases. Similarly, some antibiotics and chemotherapies can promote magnesium loss through the kidneys. Diuretics can often lead to an increased excretion of magnesium due to the corresponding water loss. Perhaps this is how magnesium deficiency often develops during alcoholism when magnesium intake is also very low due to poor nutrition.

About two thirds of all kidney stones are calcium oxalate stones. The formation of these stones is promoted by both magnesium deficiency and excessive calcium. Magnesium supplementation can hinder the development of oxalate stones by improving the solubility of magnesium oxalate and perhaps by preventing the formation of oxalate at the cellular level.

Magnesium and athletic performance

The situation where serum magnesium decreases during periods of intense activity (or when recreational athletes exert themselves beyond normal levels) is well known in sports medicine. This occurs as a result of perspiration and due to the uptake of magnesium from the bloodstream by active muscle cells. This promotes muscle cramping and decreases muscle output.

Magnesium supplementation over the course of several days has been reported to lower the occurrence of muscle cramps and strains during competitions. Several days are required for serum magnesium levels to normalize, in the absence of magnesium supplementation, following a competition.

Miscellaneous information

Magnesium deficiency is relatively common among infants primarily due to their increased requirements during growth, and also because their low body weight has not enabled the build-up of reserves. Deficiency among children can lead to cramping, nervousness and an increase in tendon reflexes and muscle tone. According to their age, daily supplementation should not exceed 100-200 mg and should only be carried out for long periods if magnesium levels are monitored. Elevated magnesium levels over longer periods can disturb bone growth in children.

Diabetics often have a magnesium deficiency which is probably caused by increased excretion from the kidneys. Magnesium deficiency may lead to complications in the later stages of diabetes.

Magnesium supplementation has been reported in the treatment of osteoporosis (especially when painful calcium phosphate deposits form during fluoride treatment). Magnesium has also been used to reduce calcification near joints after hip replacement surgery.

Magnesium deficiency has been observed alongside liver cirrhosis. This can be traced to low magnesium diets, alcoholism, medication side effects (especially diuretics), iron deficiency, as well as secondary hyperaldosteronism.

Beneficial effects of magnesium have been reported in association with premenstrual syndrome, alcohol withdrawal, neurodermatitis, cramping in newborns, convulsions later in life, and the reduction of blood lipids/fats.

MANGANESE

The enzyme-activating element

In nature, manganese is only found in small quantities, yet for humans it is essential for life. The adult body contains about 10-40 mg of manganese.

The normal daily requirement for adolescents and adults is 3-5 mg. Various sources estimate that the intestinal absorption of manganese lies somewhere between 5-40%.

Certain food components can decrease manganese absorption. These include phosphate, calcium, and iron (when consumed in large amounts). Estrogens, on the other hand, seem to improve intestinal absorption of manganese.

Manganese is almost always bound to protein. It is a component or an activator of several metabolic enzymes. Importantly, it is the essential component of the superoxide dismutase (SOD) enzyme, which protects against free radicals. Manganese is also found in the citric acid cycle enzymes pyruvate carboxylase and malate dehydrogenase.

Manganese deficiency can be caused by low manganese content in the diet or by problems that hinder its absorption from the intestine.

The following consequences of manganese deficiency have been reported:
- disrupted sugar and protein metabolism with hypoglycemia and diabetes
- fatigue and muscle atrophy
- muscle and bone problems, with a role in osteoporosis
- infertility in women
- decreased immune function
- ear problems, especially in old age (inner ear metabolism seems to be able to handle oxygen deficiency better than trace element problems)
- increased susceptibility to allergies (low manganese can lower histamine vesicle stability and increase histamine release).

Manganese has been reported to decrease blood sugar levels among diabetics. As an antagonist to vanadium, it influences enzymes involved in cholesterol metabolism. Manganese deficiency could play a role in tardive dyskinesia, which is caused by neuroleptic medications.

Manganese continued on page 75

MANGANESE

chemical symbol **Mn**

essential trace element

Normal daily requirement: adults 3-5 (up to 8) mg, children 1-2 mg
intestinal absorption approximately 40%

Functions: metabolism of carbohydrates, protein, fats, cholesterol, thyroxine and formation of collagen (especially in bones, cartilage and skin)

component of the superoxide dismutase enzyme (SOD)

Therapeutic applications: fatigue
hypoglycemia, diabetes
muscle and bone conditions
connective tissue weakness,
including slipped discs
decreased immune function
susceptibility to allergies
tardive dyskinesia (from neuroleptics)

Negative biological effects: high intake over a long time can lead to Parkinson-like symptoms and inner organ damage

Sources: whole grain products, nuts
leafy vegetables, legumes, brewer's yeast
(hardly any found in fruit and meat)

Manganese continued from page 73

Significantly more manganese is found in blood cells compared to serum; therefore even minimal hemolysis (red blood cell disintegration) can lead to an increase in blood serum concentrations. Some bodies of water and springs are rich in manganese (> 1 mg/L). Using these waters to wash hair can leave behind traces of manganese and contribute to higher hair mineral analysis results.

Hyperimidodipeptidurea (prolidase deficiency) is a genetic disorder that was discovered in 1968. The enzyme prolidase, which breaks down protein molecules in collagen, skin and vessels, requires manganese for proper function. The disorder is characterized by mental retardation, increased susceptibility to infection, and skin changes such as slow wound healing.

A genetic defect has been found in some hereditary cases of ALS (amyotrophic lateral sclerosis), a rare and fatal neurological disorder that causes atrophy of muscle and nerve cells. The defect is in the gene encoding cytoplasmic superoxide dismutase SOD1 (SOD2 is found in the mitochondria and SOD3 is localized extracellularly). The therapeutic application of antioxidants such as vitamin E and C is being studied. Manganese metabolism is associated with some cases of ALS but the exact mechanism has not been ascertained.

After a kidney transplant, free radicals can accumulate and damage the vascular endothelium. This can cause transplant arteriosclerosis, which leads to organ rejection in 3-5% of transplant cases. The frequency of organ rejection can be significantly decreased if 200 mg of human recombinant superoxide dismutase (rhSOD) is administered to the organ intra-arterially before re-establishing circulation.

Elevated manganese intake due to manganese-rich drinking water or occupational exposure (welding of manganese steel) seldom occurs.

MOLYBDENUM

chemical symbol **Mo**

recognized as an essential element in 1953

Normal daily requirement:

50-250 μg
therapeutic dosage is also within this range

Functions:

component of several enzymes, especially
sulfite, xanthine and aldehyde oxidases

Therapeutic applications:

to treat deficiency symptoms such as:
- increased sensitivity to sulfur-treated foods
  and smog (especially among asthmatics)
- decreased mental capability*
- depression*
- dental caries*
- impotence in men*
- hair loss

Negative biological effects:

not known to occur on a nutritional basis
(perhaps through antagonism with copper)

Sources:

legumes (e.g. peas, lentils)
whole grain products
bananas, brewer's yeast
wheat germ, beef liver

* therapeutic use not firmly established

MOLYBDENUM

The oxidative detoxification element

About 20 mg of molybdenum is found in an adult body. Molybdenum-containing enzymes (sulfite, xanthine, and aldehyde oxidase) are especially important for the metabolic removal of harmful substances via oxidative detoxification. Some of these substances are by-products of metabolic reactions, while others enter the body from external sources.

Sulfite oxidase breaks down sulfur compounds into sulfate, which is not harmful to humans. However, sulfur dioxide is a key irritant in smog, which is relevant for asthmatics and anyone who is highly sensitive to foods containing sulfur (such as wine). Since sulfite destroys vitamin B1, deficiencies in molybdenum and vitamin B1 often occur together. Molybdenum deficiency also disrupts the breakdown of the sulfur-containing amino acids homocysteine and cysteine. Homocysteine is implicated in the development of arteriosclerosis. High homocysteine levels increase the risk of myocardial infarction, cerebral infarction, and Alzheimer's disease.

Xanthine oxidase is responsible for the formation of uric acid. While uric acid is associated with gout among humans (an uncomfortable illness in which excess acid builds up in joints), it also has a beneficial biological role as a free radical scavenger. This protective function could contribute to an increased life expectancy among humans. This conclusion has been supported by several statistical findings. In regions where soil molybdenum concentrations are high, people have above-average life spans. Uric acid concentrations in humans are about ten times higher than in most other mammals. Some birds with particularly long life spans similarly have high uric acid levels in their bodies.

Aldehyde oxidase is important for the breakdown of various substances that often have disruptive biological effects and can promote the development of cancer if they are not broken down (by oxidative detoxification). Aldehyde oxidase is only produced in higher quantities (induced) if substances to be broken down are present.

Inherited forms of sulfite oxidase deficiency and a combination of sulfite oxidase and xanthine dehydrogenase deficiency exist. Affected infants suffer brain atrophy and die young.

Miscellaneous molybdenum functions

Molybdenum has been reported to help with male impotence (by influencing fluorine metabolism), tooth decay and iron utilization during anemia. There is some evidence that molybdenum supports the action of estrogen, especially when estrogen levels drop during and after menopause. One study measuring vitamin and trace element levels in children identified low molybdenum levels as virtually the only factor associated with low IQ in children.

A high molybdenum intake can hinder the absorption of copper. Conversely, high copper intake leads to decreased molybdenum uptake.

At first, research reports coming from Lien Xian, a 30 square kilometer region in the Chinese province of Honan, seemed like a medical mystery. This region was surprisingly found to have the highest frequency of esophageal cancer in the world. A particularly low molybdenum concentration had been found in agricultural soils. The plant enzyme nitrate reductase requires molybdenum to function. Therefore, the plants in this region lacked sufficient nitrate reductase activity. As a result, nitrogenous fertilizers were not metabolized as expected and were converted into carcinogenic nitrosamines. The nitrosamines had a particularly strong effect because vitamin C, which protects from nitrosamine damage to a certain degree, was also sparse in this region. Dietary molybdenum supplementation was promoted to decrease the risk of cancer, although supplementing plants with molybdenum would be more appropriate.

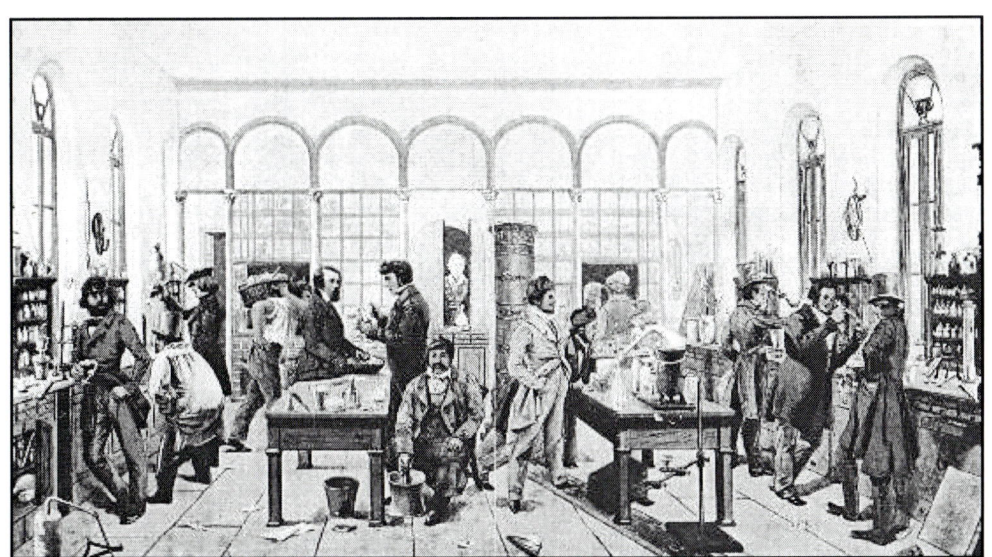

Professor Justus Von Liebig (1803-73) developed the theory of mineral nutrients in this chemistry laboratory at the University of Giessen (Germany). He added lacking minerals to soil and noted subsequent improvements in growth. His findings refuted the prevailing theory of the time that plants derived their nourishment from decayed organic matter (humus). His work led to mineral fertilizer developments and food production techniques that revolutionized agricultural and organic chemistry. This nutrient theory applies to humans as well. Humans have the potential to be healthier by providing lacking minerals in optimal concentrations.

SODIUM

Latin: *Natrium;* chemical symbol **Na**

Normal daily requirement: adults 2-3 g (4-5 g table salt)

Functions: water regulation
conduction of nerve and muscle impulses
(together with potassium)

Therapeutic applications: salt supplementation in response to high fluid
or salt loss (such as vomiting, diarrhea or
perspiration)

deficiencies due to excessive sweating
can be dangerous

Negative biological effects: high sodium can increase blood pressure

Sources: table salt
mineral water
small amounts in almost all foods

Note: high sodium levels can occur as a result
of kidney problems or excessive salt
consumption (the "hidden salt" in many foods
is problematic)

Sodium excess: for a healthy adult, consumption of over 30 g
of salt in one sitting could be life-threatening.
The vomiting reflex, however, would probably
trigger before any serious danger arose.

The difference between the daily sodium
requirement of 5 g of table salt and the lethal
dosage of 30 g may not seem that great.
However, the consequences of excess intake
are evident in cases of high blood pressure,
heart attack, and stroke. Despite these risks,
the level of public awareness remains relatively
low and few steps have been taken to limit salt
ingestion.

SODIUM

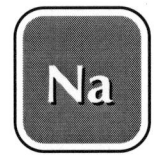

The table salt element

Sodium is abundant in nature. The earth's crust is composed of 2.6% sodium. Seawater contains almost 3% salt (sodium chloride).

Salt is found in many foods. Required by all cells in the body and found in all body fluids, sodium, in conjunction with potassium, is responsible for the origin and conduction of excitatory impulses in nerve tissues and muscles. Sufficient sodium quantities are also necessary for water regulation.

The body of an adult contains about 100 g of sodium. The daily requirement lies between 2-3 g (this corresponds to about 5 g of salt).

Even though not all details are completely understood, excessive salt consumption seems to contribute to the development of high blood pressure, which is primarily observed in industrial countries. High sodium levels have been associated with an increased risk of heart attack and stroke due to problems in the vessels of the heart and brain.

Salt was valuable in the early centuries. Salt collection and sales provided an opportunity to exploit this resource. Today, at least in industrial countries, salt use is excessive, especially when "hidden" in foods. High concentrations of salt are often used as a preservative (e.g. for fish and vegetables). Industry has taken the liberty of adding salt to food not only to add flavor, but also to add inexpensive bulk weight to mass-produced products.

For cooking purposes, it is best to use sea salt because it contains other elements such as iodine. European adults often consume 10-15 g of salt daily. Mineral water contains relatively high amounts of salt. It is recommended that patients with high blood pressure consume sodium-free water. This type of water only contains up to 20 mg/L of salt whereas regular mineral water can contain much more. Because seawater contains so much salt, anyone who is thirsty out on the ocean must never drink it. More water would be lost trying to eliminate the excess salt than could be consumed, leading to death due to dehydration.

Water decalcification systems replace excessive calcium with sodium according to the ion exchange principle. If water is very hard, sodium concentrations can be increased by 150 mg/L.

Soft drinks contain a surprisingly high amount of sodium. Cola could serve as medication in cases where diarrhea results in the loss of water and salt. While vacationing in the tropics (where diarrhea is common), soft drinks can be advantageous since they are readily available.

NICKEL

chemical symbol **Ni**

Daily requirement: could be essential for life in small quantities
toxic at higher doses

Functions: component of the urease enzyme
deficiency diseases unknown among humans
enhances the action of insulin?

Therapeutic applications: none

Negative biological effects: allergies
can damage gametes
antagonism of zinc and copper

Sources: abundant in nature (humans do not need to be
concerned about deficiencies)
- fashion jewelry (white metal)
- tobacco, cigarette smoke
- orthopedic and medical implants
- nickel refinery waste
- cosmetics and hair dyes
- chemicals

NICKEL
The fashion jewelry element

Nickel is a typical example of an element that is potentially essential to life in minute quantities, yet clearly toxic at high levels.

About 10 mg of nickel is found in an adult human. The amount of nickel absorbed daily varies between 100 and 900 µg; therefore according to current knowledge, long-term deficiency is unlikely when following a normal diet.

Small amounts of nickel seem to be required for the proper function of some thyroid and adrenal gland hormones. Nickel seems to enhance the action of insulin, lessen the effect of adrenaline and influence fat metabolism and blood fat content. In 1995, nickel was identified as a component of the urease enzyme (which breaks down urea). Two nickel atoms are required in the active center of the urease enzyme.

High nickel levels are found in patients suffering from stroke, severe burns, and sometimes cancer. Sweat contains a relatively high amount of nickel and can lead to higher hair mineral analysis results. Humans are particularly exposed to nickel through tobacco and cigarette smoke, and it can also be absorbed through the skin. Nickel is especially toxic in combination with carbon monoxide. This creates nickel carbonyl, which is oncogenic (promotes cancer) and lethal in higher quantities. Waste from nickel refineries provides another source of nickel to the environment.

Other sources of nickel include fashion jewelry made with white metal, orthopedic and medical implants, and some cosmetics and hair dyes. Direct nickel contact can lead to an allergic reaction – a common condition characterized by localized inflammation with an itchy and burning rash (contact allergy). After some time, these irritations can appear in areas other than the original point of contact. Common areas include arms, elbows, hands, face, neck, eyelids and inner thighs.

Nickel poisoning is relatively rare and virtually unknown to the medical field. The first phase involves mild and unspecific symptoms such as headaches, vomiting, nausea and excessive sweating, chest and breathing problems. The second phase starts about 12-36 hours after nickel intake, and involves chest pains followed by blue discoloration of the hands and face, as well as weakness, increased body temperature and lung inflammation (similar to a viral lung inflammation). Serious poisoning can result in death within 4-11 days due to edema in the lungs or brain, or due to damage of the liver, spleen, kidneys or adrenal glands.

PHOSPHOROUS

chemical symbol **P**

essential for life

Normal daily requirement: 0.7-0.8 g

Functions:

energy metabolism
bone development
teeth

Therapeutic applications:

phosphorous deficiency should not be a concern with normal diets since it is present in all foods

frequent addition of phosphate should be discouraged

Negative biological effects:

behavior disorders in children (ADD/ADHD) may be linked to high levels of phosphorous (found as an additive in foodstuffs)

Sources:

in all foods, especially fish, meat, poultry, eggs, whole grain products, nuts, soft drinks, and soft ice cream

Phosphate deficiency:

a deficiency in the diet can remain unnoticed for a long time since phosphorous can be mobilized from bone deposits. Phosphate deficiency often occurs in areas affected by famine (for example, in Germany during and after World War II). It can also occur due to disturbances in kidney function, vitamin D deficiency, and over-activity of the parathyroid gland. Symptoms of phosphate deficiency include muscle weakness and softening of the bones. Protein deficiency often exists simultaneously.

PHOSPHOROUS

Important for energy and bone structure

Phosphorous is found in all cells of the body. ATP molecules (used in energy metabolism) contain phosphorus. It is also found as a component of lecithin in membranes of nerve cells in particular. In mineral form, it is an important structural component of bones and teeth. The body of an adult contains about 1 kg of phosphorous. Many of its functions require the presence of calcium, magnesium and vitamin D. Since phosphorous is absorbed across the intestinal wall into the blood twice as efficiently as calcium, our diet should contain less phosphorous than calcium (at a ratio of approximately 1:1.5).

The intestine absorbs about 60% of the phosphorous contained in food (in infants this can be as high as 90%). The proportion absorbed rises when less phosphorous is available or when the body's requirement increases. Absorption is enhanced by vitamin D and hindered by iron, aluminum, calcium and phytate.

The excretion of phosphorous is regulated by parathyroid gland hormones and takes place primarily via the kidneys. Excretion can be increased marginally by estrogen and thyroxine, and decreased by insulin, growth hormone and cortisol. Elevated phosphorous excretion can lead to the formation of phosphate-containing kidney stones.

The best natural sources are fish, meat, poultry, eggs, whole grain products and nuts. People following a normal diet rarely develop long-term deficiencies. However, many people may be consuming too much phosphorous, especially from sausages, industrially produced food, processed cheese, cola, and drinks that are preserved by the addition of phosphates.

Pregnant women, heavy laborers, and top athletes may require higher amounts of dietary phosphorous.

Some reports associate behavior/attention and academic problems in children (especially ADD/ADHD) with elevated phosphorous levels. A low phosphate diet (not absolutely phosphate-free) has apparently helped some of these children. The beneficial effects may be due to a reduction in consumption of industrially processed food (including food colorings and other chemical additives that can also induce allergic responses). Children following this diet often eat food with a higher nutritional value, including trace elements and vitamins, and less refined sugar.

LEAD

Latin: *Plumbum,* chemical symbol **Pb**

poisonous ☠

Functions:
none known (poisonous mineral)
also toxic to animals and plants

Therapeutic applications:
none

Negative biological effects:
Typical poisoning symptoms are:
- weakness, "leadened" fatigue
- depression, sleep disturbances
- anemia, pallor
- indigestion, colic, kidney damage
- bone pain
- blood vessel spasms accompanied by nausea and disturbances in vision and hearing
- nerve damage, particularly in the optic nerve (leading to blindness)
- brain damage in children
- behavioral and mental disturbances

Sources:
paints, print colors and rust protectant
leaded gasoline, automobile emissions
lead batteries, leaded glass
lead alloys, old water pipes

Note:
Factors that protect against toxicity:
- zinc, selenium, calcium, magnesium
- sulfur-containing amino acids
- vitamins A, C, E and B-complex

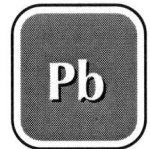

LEAD

The toxic element in automobile emissions (leaded gas)

Lead is actually a very rare element. It is found at an average concentration of only 0.02 ppm within the earth's crust. In contrast, cobalt and molybdenum, which are essential for human life, are even rarer than lead. Since ores with a high lead content are quite common, lead has been well known since antiquity. Water pipes in ancient Rome were made of up to 99.3% lead. This illustrates how efficient the Romans were at lead mining and processing. Lead was also present in glazes and therefore often used at the tables of wealthy Romans. Since chronic lead poisoning can diminish physical ability, the military might of the Romans (especially those of higher rank) may have been weakened by lead poisoning, contributing to the downfall of the Roman Empire.

Lead was used as a material for water pipes until the beginning of the 20th century. Its burden on the environment has been increasing as a result of the enormous production of leaded gasoline since 1921 when lead's anti-knocking properties were discovered. The lead content of Greenland's snow masses can be used as an indicator of the degree of ambient environmental lead pollution. From 1750 to 1950, the amount of lead in Greenland's snow masses was 10 mg/kg, but today it is 210 mg/kg. Therefore, lead pollution has risen sharply in the last century.

In the US, about 400,000 children between ages 1 and 5 become ill from lead poisoning every year (according to Daunderer 1994). Paints that contain lead cause most of these cases! The impacts are considerable, and include anemia and behavior/mental disturbance.

Studies in the US have shown that higher blood concentrations in children have been statistically correlated with an increase in behavior problems (such as aggressiveness, delinquency, and criminal offences) and physical complaints.

Absorption of large quantities of lead compounds within a short period of time leads to acute poisoning. Damage to muscle, nervous and kidney tissue can cause cramps, paralysis and even death. Lab values above 70-80 µg Pb^{2+} per 100 ml of whole blood indicate acute lead poisoning and the need for immediate medical treatment. Since blood cells contain about ten times more lead than serum, even slight hemolysis can falsely elevate blood serum concentrations.

Sub-acute lead poisoning can exist when lead values are slightly lower than in acute cases. Symptoms include fatigue, loss of appetite, gastric complaints and headaches.

Lead toxicity should be considered when the following combination of symptoms presents: joint pain without inflammation, muscle tension (especially back muscles), spastic intractable constipation, skin pallor and psychological disturbances.

Severe symptoms are unlikely when blood values are below 30 µg. In 1996, the German Human Biomonitoring Commission reported that 1% of all children and 1.6% of women in their childbearing ages have blood lead concentrations over 10 µg/100 ml. Of the remaining adults, 1.5% has lead levels over 15 µg/100 ml. Since lead acts in very small amounts but affects humans over a prolonged period of time, chronic lead poisoning should still be considered due to lead's action on the nerves and brain. This is especially applicable to pregnant women and small children. In the US, it is normal to perform blood analyses on children with learning difficulties, behavioral problems and/or prior to starting psychotherapy. Studies in New Zealand (1993) and Australia (1992) have indicated that delayed infant development, prolonged deficits in attention and mental performance, and a decrease in IQ levels by 4-5% have occurred in some regions where there is high lead exposure. Although hardly noticeable at the individual level, lead poisoning can damage the economic stability and potential of a region.

Damage caused by lead typically affects the blood and kidneys. Kidney impairment often causes high blood pressure. Disturbances in the formation of hemoglobin lead to the appearance of urinary metabolites such as aminolavulinic acid (ALA) and porphyrines. Lead toxicity in adults, leading to urinary excretion of more than 6 mg ALA/L, is associated with psychological complaints such as depression, exhaustion and sleep/concentration disturbances.

Lead has been observed to interfere with the production of several hormones and with the production of sperm in the testes. Further reports indicate the damaging effects of lead on chromosomes – which can promote cancer development.

Lead is partly deposited in bones and can be mobilized in response to infections or certain medications (cortisone in particular!). This release can result in the sudden appearance of lead poisoning symptoms, which may be overlooked if they are masked by the symptoms of the current illness (causing problems for diagnosis and therapy).

Besides anemia, the main cause of the grayish skin pallor observed with lead toxicity is the constriction of small vessels within the skin. When toxicity becomes worse, a blue lining may appear along the gums, often accompanied by flat precipitates on the mucosal tissue of the lips, cheeks and tongue.

Due to the increased accumulation of lead in our environment over the last few decades, the risk of chronic lead toxicity for everyone rises with age. Lead is accumulating in the food chain through the use of pesticides. Many people have not noticed that portions of their residential plumbing system or pipes leading to their homes, in place since the 19th century, are made of lead. Lead pipes are found in 10-20% of homes in Germany. This type of heavy metal exposure can lead to the development of a new illness, or worsen an existing illness – particularly if the heavy metal toxicity and the illness affect the same organ or enzymatic pathway. It is impossible to completely avoid lead, no matter how hard we try. Lead poisoning due to occupational exposure may be covered by worker's compensation.

PLATINUM

chemical symbol **Pt**

poisonous ☠

Functions:
none known
poisonous when taken up by the body

Therapeutic applications:
platinum compound Cisplatin is used in cancer treatment as a cytotoxic agent

Negative biological effects:
allergies affecting airways
lung cancer
leukemia
fatigue
eczema

Sources:
catalytic converter
photography paper
metal and platinum processing industry

Factors that protect against platinum:
- beta-carotene, vitamins C and E
- selenium, zinc, manganese, copper
- free radical scavengers

To reduce the danger of platinum:
- avoid poorly ventilated parking garages, especially below ground level;
- close the outside vents of the car in heavy traffic;
- take antioxidants as a preventive measure to minimize free radical reactions (beta-carotene, vitamins C and E, selenium, zinc, manganese).

The serum concentration of lipid peroxides is an indication of the presence and quantity of free radicals. An increased antioxidant intake should be considered if these levels are high.

PLATINUM

Pt

The poisonous element in catalytic converters

Platinum is one of the rarest elements on earth. It forms only $5 \times 10^{-7}\%$ of the earth's crust. Platinum is a precious metal.

The catalytic converter of a car, containing about 0.5-2 g of platinum (alone or as an alloy), is the most important and most interesting of all platinum sources. Under average driving conditions, about 50,000 billion (5×10^{13}) platinum atoms are released, corresponding to a platinum production of 0.8-1.6 mg per 1000 km driving distance.

The maximum allowable workplace concentration is 2 µg per cubic meter of air. In the catalytic converter, platinum enables free radical reactions. This may be good for the environment, but the fine platinum dust blown out can have negative biological consequences. The finer the dust, the deeper it penetrates the airways, eventually reaching the alveoli of the lungs.

Free radicals produce chain reactions which are dangerous to living cells. Cell damage occurs through the peroxidation of unsaturated fats, including those in cellular membranes. Damage also occurs through enzyme activation and the alteration of nucleic acid structures.

Platinum that comes in contact with the alveoli (where the blood takes up oxygen) has been associated with an increased incidence of lung cancer and leukemia. In the US, a significant rise in lung cancer was found following the introduction of the catalytic converter.

Photography students in Chicago who came into contact with platinum-containing photography paper experienced airway allergies similar to those of platinum refinery workers. In Sweden, serious sensitivity reactions to complex platinum salts were observed among workers in metal processing refineries. They developed eczema on their hands, eye irritation, a constrictive feeling in the chest, and extreme fatigue by the end of the workday.

Platinum stays in the body for a long time since it dwells in organs that are rich in fats, including the adrenal gland. Platinum in this area can damage the hormonal system. Even the immune system can be damaged, possibly diminishing the body's ability to defend itself against infections.

Platinum can react with several amino acids to form complex compounds, such as cisplatin – a cytotoxic agent used in cancer therapy. The actions and side effects of cytotoxic agents are primarily based on free radical reactions, as is the case with cisplatin. As a chemical, cisplatin has been known since 1845.

SULFUR

chemical symbol **S**

Normal daily requirement: not clear (0.5-1 g*)
* amount is not clearly defined because sufficient protein consumption usually ensures adequate sulfur uptake

Functions: component of sulfur-containing amino acids and therefore found in almost all proteins

especially important for:
- detoxification functions in the liver
- connective tissue of skin, hair and joints

Therapeutic applications: liver and connective tissue support
external application to skin and hair

Negative biological effects: only in the form of chemicals

Sources: meat
fish
eggs

SULFUR
Used for centuries to treat skin conditions

Sulfur is a structural component of the amino acids cysteine, homocysteine, methionine and taurine, also known as the sulfur amino acids. Sulfur is found in practically all proteins. Its significance includes its ability to form disulfide (S-S) bridges between different parts of a molecule or between different protein chains. Sulfur is therefore an important structural component of connective and supporting tissues. Sulfur is mostly found in the skin, nails, hair (in the form of keratin) and joints. Adequate sulfur intake is often recommended whenever there is an illness involving these areas. Sulfur has been used for centuries in ointments and tinctures to treat skin conditions.

The liver contains a relatively high amount of sulfur, which is important for detoxification functions. Many poisonous substances and metabolic by-products are detoxified in the liver with the help of sulfur in its activated sulfate form. They are then made water-soluble, facilitating excretion by the kidneys into the urine. The sulfur compound Dimercaprol is used to treat heavy metal poisoning.

The best natural sources of sulfur are meat, fish and eggs. Sulfur deficiencies are almost impossible if sufficient protein is taken in. General sulfur deficiencies are not described due to the inevitable simultaneous protein deficiency – the protein deficiency is more important and producing more problems than the sulfur deficiency. Similarly, excess protein consumption with simultaneous excess sulfur ingestion has not been identified.

Some foods such as dried fruits and wine (which only picks up the taste of sulfur if levels exceed 50 mg/L) are preserved by sulfation. This can lead to side effects among sensitive individuals (headaches, nausea, dizziness).

Some sulfur chemicals such as H_2S and CS_2 smell like rotten eggs. Some people may be familiar with this smell from chemistry class. These chemicals are poisonous, although one would hardly come into contact with them in everyday life.

The combustion of coal, oil, gas, and wood produces a large amount of sulfur dioxide (SO_2), which is harmful for humans and the environment. It is dispersed by air and often travels great distances. Sulfur dioxide is well known for its role in the destruction of forests and lakes due to acid rain in regions far away from the origin of pollution. As a component of smog, sulfur dioxide is also damaging to the bronchi.

ANTIMONY

Latin: *Stibium*; chemical symbol **Sb**

poisonous ☠

Functions:	no known body function (poisonous)
Therapeutic applications:	found in some medications that are used to treat tropical illnesses
Negative biological effects:	usually occur secondary to industrial exposure excessive skin production and pigmentation nerve damage
Sources:	almost exclusively industrial

ANTIMONY

The poisonous element of centuries past

Antimony compounds have been known since antiquity. They are now used in alloys, fireworks and matches, in the manufacturing of paper and as a preparatory agent in the dye industry.

When taken up in the bloodstream, antimony compounds are almost as toxic as arsenic compounds yet they are absorbed much more poorly from the intestines. Because they also cause serious irritation to mucosal tissues, they are often rejected and expelled by vomiting.

Acute poisoning is recognized by gastric complaints (cramps, vomiting and diarrhea) as well as headaches and nausea. This can lead to muscle twitching, disturbed kidney and brain function and ultimately coma.

Prolonged intake of small amounts can lead to chronic poisoning. This is characterized by excessive skin formation (hyperkeratosis) on the hands and feet, skin pigmentation and nerve damage (polyneuropathy). Nerve damage begins with sensitivity disturbances and evolves into paralysis.

Centuries ago, antimony was medicinally used to induce vomiting and to encourage the expulsion of bronchial phlegm.

Today, organic antimony compounds are still used in remedies to treat tropical illnesses such as schistosomiasis, loaiasis, and trichimoniasis.

SELENIUM

chemical symbol **Se**

recognized as an **essential** element in 1957

Normal daily requirement:
50-200 µg or 1-1.5 µg/kg body weight
optimally 250-300 µg
temporary therapeutic doses of up to 1 mg

Functions:
component of glutathione peroxidase
component of an enzyme required for
thyroxine production (discovered in 1991)

protects from free radicals, x-rays and
chromosome damage

stimulates immune defenses, including an
increased germ resistance

Therapeutic applications:
autoimmune disease, AIDS, cancer,
chronic infection, and inflammation

muscle disease (including heart attacks)

liver disease (including alcoholism)

pancreatitis, diabetes

deterring platelet aggregation

heavy metal poisoning (especially
mercury and cadmium)

free radicals: "diseases of civilization,
degenerative conditions (cataracts,
glaucoma, aging, osteoarthritis or joint
degeneration), and radiation damage

Negative biological effects:
selenosis has occurred in some
South American regions after prolonged
intake of over 2-4 mg/day

Sources:
whole grain products, including rice
fish, meat, milk

SELENIUM

Se

The versatile element with anti-oxidant properties

From a scientific standpoint, selenium has had an eventful history. Discovered in 1817, it was first used medicinally in the treatment of inoperable tumors, where it was surprisingly successful. In the 1930's and 1940's it was deemed to be extremely poisonous, and often was mistaken for arsenic. Intensive research began worldwide on a larger scale after 1957, when it was proven that selenium is essential to human life.

Selenium preparations have been used routinely in veterinary medicine for a long time, and not only for the infamous selenium deficiency disease of lambs – the "white muscle disease." Selenium's therapeutic benefit to humans is rarely recognized, however it has been used extensively in several countries. As a result of governmental decisions in Finland, selenium has been added to grain since 1984.

The adult human body contains about 10-30 mg of selenium. The highest concentrations are found in the kidneys, glands, liver, blood platelets, and in the lens of the eye. The daily requirement for adults is 50-200 µg (250-300 µg is optimal). The minimum requirement is estimated to be at least 1 µg/kg of body weight. 50-75% of selenium contained in salts is absorbed in the intestine, while the absorption of selenium from organic compounds is 100%. In some cases, up to 1 mg doses have been applied therapeutically (individual cases have exceeded this amount). Some regions on earth have high selenium content in their soils. Even though poisoning symptoms can be expected among sensitive people taking prolonged daily doses of 2 mg, people living in these areas have been tolerating 3 mg/day for prolonged periods of time without complications.

Selenium poisoning symptoms are referred to as selenosis, and include gastric problems, irritability, fatigue, headaches, disturbances in hair and nail growth accompanied by brittle fingernails and hair loss, and a characteristic garlic-like breath odor (caused by the elimination of selenium compounds through the lungs).

In principle, selenium is consumed by humans following absorption from the soil by plants. These plants may then be consumed by other animals. Plants usually do not require selenium. However, selenium can be utilized by plants in metabolic processes in place of sulfur. Plant sources are the main way that animals and humans get selenium.

Many regions were washed out to a great extent during the Ice Ages thus reducing the selenium content of these soils. Remaining selenium compounds become insoluble due to acid rain, hindering their ability to be absorbed by plants. Also, environmental pollution alters the acidity of soil and deposits heavy metals (in considerable amounts) into the soil. These heavy metals react with selenium to form insoluble compounds.

Heart attacks and Big-joint disease

Human selenium deficiency diseases that occurred in the Chinese province of Keshan include Keshan disease and big-joint disease. In the Chinese province of Keshan (population of ~50 million), up to 10% of the population had been dying of heart failure over many decades. This included a high proportion of young children, adolescents and young women. Eventually, the main cause was determined to be heart damage (and decreased immunity) due to selenium deficiency. Viral infection in the end stages often resulted in accelerated death. Today, the people in this region are obligated to take a 1 mg selenium tablet each week. As a result of this large-scale administration, Keshan disease has almost been eradicated.

In the same region, an illness known as "big-joint disease" exists (named after the monstrous joint swelling that occurs). In some villages, the illness was so common that fruit was left unpicked because nobody could climb the trees. Selenium deficiency was also identified as a major factor contributing to this illness. X-ray results surprisingly confirmed that selenium intake improved arthrotic conditions.

While Keshan and big-joint diseases may seem exotic, the importance of selenium in heart disease remains clear. Unfortunately, it is not widely known that selenium deficiency increases the likelihood of heart attack (myocardial infarction). This fact was established through research conducted primarily in Finland (also in New Zealand and Germany). Finland once had the highest incidence of heart attacks in Europe, even though this country is certainly not stressed by politics. Finnish people tend to be healthy thanks to their saunas. Selenium deficiency in this country can be considered a cause, or at least a significant factor in the increase in heart attack risk. Soils in this region were severely depleted of selenium when they were washed out during the Ice-Age. Now, selenium levels in Finland are becoming further diminished by acid rain coming from middle Europe (which has also contributed to biologically dead lakes in northern Europe).

The government of Finland began a selenium campaign in 1984, which involved increasing public awareness, selenium fertilization of soils and the obligatory addition of selenium to grain.

The use of fertilizers that contain sulfur, such as ammonium sulfate, hinders the ability of plants to absorb selenium and should therefore be avoided.

Unfortunately, the success observed in Finland goes almost unnoticed in other countries. Perhaps if the incidence of heart attacks decreased due to selenium supplementation, waiting lists for coronary by-pass operations would not be as long (sometimes these waiting periods are fatal to patients). After all, selenium treatment is a much cheaper alternative to surgery, and cheaper than the cost of heart medication used following the operation. Selenium deficiency increases the tendency of platelets to aggregate, which also plays a role in heart attacks. Blood thinning drugs have been used for many years to prevent to occurrence (or recurrence) of heart attacks. For these patients, plasma selenium levels should be 60 µg/L (versus the 20 µg/L seen in among Keshan patients) to obtain a protective effect.

Pancreatitis

The list of diseases associated with selenium deficiency (which are treated by therapeutic selenium supplementation) has continued to grow. For example, in 1993 a large clinic in Germany reported that immediate selenium treatment prevented patients from dying of acute pancreatitis – a relatively rare yet often fatal disease. The following sections describe other important areas for possible therapeutic selenium use.

Cancer and the immune system

Extensive literature concerning selenium and the development of cancer dates back to 1920, when Watson-Williams successfully treated 72 inoperable cancer patients with colloidal selenium. Eight of these patients were reported to have completely recovered. Many examples provide evidence that selenium inhibits cancers of the skin, liver, lung, breast and intestine.

In other countries, selenium deficiency is regarded as an increased risk factor in the development of cancer. Vitamin E deficiency is considered to further increase this risk.

It is generally known that cytostatic treatment weakens the immune system, allowing otherwise minor disease agents to become life threatening. Some medical practitioners do not know that cytostatic treatment often leads to selenium deficiency.

Selenium supplementation can diminish the toxic side effects of cytostatic treatment without compromising therapeutic benefits.

Animal research has shown that selenium supplementation can decrease the damaging effects of the drugs Adriamycin and Cisplatin on the heart and kidney, respectively. Some patients who did not respond to cytostatic treatment improved after selenium was incorporated into the treatment. Therefore, a daily selenium supplement of 100-300 µg is often recommended for cancer patients.

The possibility of selenium deficiency should be considered in cases of aberrant immune function. Individual reports cite the role of selenium in hemolytic anemia, cardiomyopathy, chronic infection, and even in multiple sclerosis (research by the Danish MS Society).

Selenium and AIDS

One of the main factors in the rapid spread of AIDS, in addition to sexual and other activity, is the deficiency of selenium from our soils, food and water. In African countries with selenium-rich soils there is a lower incidence of AIDS. Current information on selenium and AIDS is described in the book *What Really Causes AIDS* by Professor Harold D Foster.

Selenium and rheumatic diseases

Prolonged selenium supplementation in China has reduced the incidence of "big-joint disease" in children from 42% to 4% in areas where this illness was common. Various other illnesses of rheumatic nature have been successfully treated with selenium, in addition to vitamin E and several other vitamins and trace elements. In some cases, high selenium doses (1 mg) have resolved symptoms that persisted for years.

Glutathione peroxidase and arteriosclerosis

Selenium is a component of glutathione peroxidase, an enzyme found in almost every cell. This enzyme is particularly abundant in red blood cells and is found primarily in platelets, phagocytes, liver cells and retinal cells. It is composed of four identical subunits, each containing one atom of selenium. Because glutathione peroxidase is active in the cytoplasm, its antioxidative effects are considered about 1000 times stronger than those of the fat soluble antioxidant vitamin E. Selenium is a significant protective and defensive factor against free radicals and oxidative damage from both external (radiation and environmental toxins) and internal sources (metabolic by-products). Its effects on arachidonic acid and prostaglandin metabolism in platelets are well documented. Selenium deficiency plays a significant role in the development of arteriosclerosis, including coronary heart disease (where we are increasingly finding chronic inflammation as a major pathogenic factor). Heart muscle cells seem to have special proteins that contain selenium; this is an area of continuing research.

Selenium and thyroid hormone

A selenium-containing enzyme responsible for the production of thyroid hormone was discovered in 1991. Therefore, selenium deficiency in addition to iodine deficiency can contribute to diminished thyroid hormone production (leading to thyroid problems such as goiter). It is possible that both selenium and iodine deficiencies can have simultaneous effects in some cases (more about this in the iodine chapter).

Free radicals, SOD, and neuropsychiatric disease

Free radicals play an important role in many diseases, especially in chronic illnesses that are considered degenerative and/or rheumatic in nature. Some brain researchers are studying the significance of free radicals in Alzheimer's and Parkinson's diseases and in amyotrophic lateral sclerosis (ALS; Lou Gehrig's disease). In 1993, an autosomal dominant genetic defect, which disrupts the function of superoxide dismutase SOD1, was found to cause ALS. Treatment with antioxidants is being studied.

In 1994, an antioxidant (Freedox) was approved in Austria to treat subarachnoid bleeding in the brain – a rare but often fatal condition. Freedox is advertised as the first antioxidant to prevent progressive secondary damage, support the protective mechanism of nerve cells, stabilize cellular membranes and maintain their vitamin E content. One vial of the infusion (100 ml with 150 mg of the active ingredient) costs approximately $115 USD.

In 1994, a transplant center in Munich reported that superoxide dismutase (given intra-arterially as 200 mg of rhSOD; rh = recombinant human) could significantly improve the long-term rejection rate of kidney transplants (by lessening organ-damaging vessel reactions caused by free radicals after reperfusion).

Alcohol and liver cirrhosis

It has been noted that blood fats or cholesterol only become problematic for blood vessel walls (arteriosclerosis) after they have been altered by free radicals and peroxides. This also seems to play an important role in the development of liver cirrhosis among alcoholics, since alcohol influences liver metabolism leading to an increased production of peroxides. Due to the poor selenium content of alcoholic beverages and the unhealthy diet followed by many alcoholics, selenium-dependent protective mechanisms are ineffective.

Miscellaneous indications for selenium

- patients on kidney dialysis;
- serious infection (especially after surgery);
- serious burns;
- after long periods of fasting;
- people on restrictive diets (seniors);
- pregnancy or infancy (periods with an increased need for selenium).

Selenium also plays an important role in the detoxification of various heavy metals, especially mercury and cadmium.

SILICON

chemical symbol **Si**

essential for life

Normal daily requirement: not clear (20-200 mg)
only 1-4 % is absorbed in the intestine

Functions: elasticity and stability of connective tissue in:
- bones
- skin
- blood vessels

deposition of minerals within bones

enhances activity of white blood cells in the immune system

Therapeutic applications: corresponding body functions for connective tissue and skin problems

Negative biological effects: prolonged exposure to silicon dust can lead to silicosis of the lung

Sources: whole grain products
fruits and vegetables

SILICON
The element for skin, hair, nails, and more

Silicon is the second most abundant chemical element (25%) in the earth's crust aside from oxygen (50%). Plants require silicon for photosynthesis and it is also an essential trace element for humans. Many antacids contain silicon compounds (silicates). Silica (SiO_2) is the most frequently used form of silicon in nutritional supplements.

An adult human body contains about 1 g of silicon. Silicon is necessary for the formation of the structural protein collagen. Collagen is found within the connective tissue of blood vessels, skin, hair, cartilage, and especially in bone. It is important for elasticity and strength. Within the bones, silicon also encourages the deposition of minerals (a positive type of calcification) on a pre-existing protein scaffold.

Silicon accumulates within the mitochondria of osteoblasts, where it is required for the optimal function of the enzyme prolylhydroxylase. Prolylhydroxylase activity is regarded as an indicator of the rate of collagen biosynthesis. Collagen synthesis also requires vitamin C to some extent (in the construction of hexosamines).

In the immune system, silica stimulates the activity of white blood cells.

In general, plant foods are relatively rich in silicon.

Silicon deposits in the spleen and liver have been found repeatedly among patients with kidney failure (uremia, with and without dialysis). Healthy people likely excrete a certain amount of silicon through the kidneys.

If silicon is consumed in the form of a colloidal gel, no medications, vitamins or trace elements should be taken for the next four hours. Similar to activated charcoal, the gel (which is only absorbed in the intestine in small amounts) absorbs many substances leading to their elimination. This can be favorable if the substances are harmful or toxic. To avoid interference with the absorption of useful substances, it is best to take silicon gel before going to bed.

Silicosis is a relatively common occupational illness. Long-term inhalation of quartz or silicon dust leads to extensive changes in the lungs due to increased production of connective tissue. This is especially common in mining and in areas where cutting and sand blasting is performed without protective masks. About 100 years ago, silicosis among miners reached tragic frequencies. Today, its occurrence has significantly decreased due to protective measures. Routine screening can identify silicosis at an early stage.

TIN

Latin: *Stannum*; chemical symbol **Sn**

Normal daily requirement:
unclear for humans
toxic in larger amounts
the average diet provides about 2-3 mg daily

Functions:
unclear for humans

component of gastrin, which stimulates the production of gastric acid

deficiency symptoms have only been identified in animals

dietary tin deficiency in humans has not been reported

Negative biological effects:
mild to severe poisoning symptoms

Sources:
- dental fillings (which contain other heavy metals such as mercury)
- poor quality tin cans without protective inner coatings

TIN

The trace element with unclear importance

Tin was frequently used in antiquity, especially in metal alloys. This included bronzes (copper and tin alloys), bearing metals and soldering metals. Due to its stability in damp and humid conditions, it was often used to plate other metals. Because of its malleability, tin can be pressed into thin sheets ("stanniol") at room temperature.

Today, tin cans are almost always lined with a protective inner coating due to the risk of tin poisoning. When tin cans are left open, time, high storage temperatures and acidity promote the release of tin into the contents. Acute poisoning can develop, accompanied by vomiting, stomach aches, diarrhea and headaches. The relatively low absorption rate of tin compounds in the intestine provides a certain degree of protection against poisoning. The contents of tin cans should be transferred to porcelain or glass dishes immediately after opening. The release of tin and other heavy metals can be checked by looking for black/gray discolorations on the inside surfaces of empty cans.

Little is known about tin's biological activity in humans. It seems to be a component of gastrin, which stimulates the production of gastric acid. Tin might be exclusively essential to animals. After one to two weeks, animals on tin-free diets exhibit deficiency symptoms of delayed growth, hair loss and suppressed appetite.

The average diet provides humans with about 2-3 mg of tin daily. A daily requirement level has not been identified since tin has not been shown to be essential in humans, nor has there been any mention of human deficiency diseases or essential metabolic functions involving tin.

In some occupations, lung disease has occurred due to the inhalation of vapors containing tin.

Some highly poisonous organic tin compounds are used as stabilizers in plastics and disinfectants, and as antifungal agents. Some of these tin compounds are used to protect the hulls of ships. While in transit, these ships release poison directly into the ocean. Sadly, an incident involving poisonous organic tin exposure in France led to the deaths of 110 people in 1954.

STRONTIUM

chemical symbol **Sr**

Normal daily requirement: no daily requirement

Functions: no significant functions known
at the present time

Therapeutic applications: none, except for radioactive Sr-90 in
radiation therapy

Negative biological effects: within the body, strontium is absorbed by
bones in place of calcium, especially during
calcium deficiency

Sources: found with the other alkali earth elements
calcium and magnesium (and barium)

radioactive strontium-90 is formed by nuclear
weapon explosions and reactor accidents
such as Chernobyl

STRONTIUM
Used for radiation therapy and nuclear weapons

After magnesium and calcium, strontium is the third (and barium is the fourth) alkali earth element. In nature, it is almost always found in small amounts in association with other elements of this group.

In medicine, the naturally occurring isotopes Sr-84, 86 and 87 are used in bone scans while the radioactive isotopes Sr-89 and 90 are applied for radiation therapy. In 1998, reports described the use of radioactive strontium-89 in the treatment of cancer pain, especially in patients with bone metastases of prostate carcinoma.

Individual reports have noted that organisms might require strontium in trace amounts. According to current research, deficiencies leading to negative effects rarely arise since small amounts of strontium are found almost everywhere in nature.

Technical applications of strontium include its use as a red light source in the production of fireworks and signal lights. It was previously used in the manufacture of electronic circuits.

Sadly, strontium is famous for its association with atomic bombs (especially from testing in the 1950's and 1960's) and nuclear reactor accidents (even before Chernobyl). Elevated amounts of strontium-90 were released, increasing the risk of bone marrow damage. It was a major component of the radioactive fallout that remained a concern for many years after these catastrophes. In this respect, strontium-90 is as worrisome as radioactive iodine and cobalt. The formation of radioactive cobalt for weapons use led to the term "cobalt bomb!" The long-term consequences of possessing atomic bombs are detrimental even to countries on the offensive.

The Calcium connection

In both its normal and radioactive forms, strontium can act synergistically with calcium in some cases, and antagonistically to it at other times.

Like calcium, strontium is deposited in bones. In calcium deficiency, which leads to osteoporosis, increased amounts of other elements are absorbed by the bones. Strontium (as well as lead and cadmium) is particularly absorbed in calcium-deficient states. Conversely, strontium absorption can be significantly decreased by calcium supplementation.

THALLIUM

chemical symbol **Tl**

poisonous ☠

Functions: extremely poisonous

effective rat poison

Therapeutic applications: none known

Negative biological effects: psychological disturbance is reported in case studies from Heidelberg-Emmertsgrund where thallium pollution was identified much too late

Sources: industrial waste
rat poison

manufacturing of synthetic gemstones, special glass, and fluorescent color

THALLIUM

The element in rat poison and industrial waste

Thallium is released into the environment through its use in rat poison and the manufacture of special glass, fluorescent colors and synthetic gemstones. Thallium poisoning is associated with these environmental exposures.

Thallium poisoning begins mildly and involves nausea, vomiting and diarrhea, followed by a symptom-free period of 2-3 days. After this, serious gastric illness (vomiting and diarrhea) re-appears accompanied by kidney damage. As poisoning progresses, nerve damage develops (toxic polyneuropathy) which affects the legs in particular. A complete loss of hair is characteristic and occurs after the 13 day of poisoning at the earliest. Pubic and underarm hair may also be affected. In less severe cases, general hair loss may be the only noticeable symptom. After 3-4 weeks, vertical stripes of a half-moon shape typically appear on fingernails and toenails.

Thallium salts are absorbed well in the intestine and tend to accumulate in hair and skin. With a half-life of 14 days, they are eventually excreted through the kidney and intestinal tract. Poisoning can also affect animals – for example, if cats eat rats that have been poisoned by thallium.

An incident in 1988 still serves as a cautionary reminder today. The media published the headlines "Soviet children suffer from environmental illness" and described an illness that affected about 120 children in one Soviet province. Beginning with flu-like symptoms and hallucinations and ending with hair loss, this illness brought panic to the Russian city of Tschernowizy. Thallium poisoning was eventually identified and acid rain in the region was suspected to be the cause. Fortunately, all children recovered completely.

Heidelberg-Emmertsgrund is a relatively well-known residential area in Germany – only 4 miles from the city of Leimen where the tennis star Boris Becker was born. Many years ago, the industrial wastes of a nearby concrete plant had been deposited in Heidelberg-Emmertsgrund. Frequent large-scale psychological disturbances, including high suicide rates, were observed in this area. Alexander Mitscherlich, a renowned psychologist, conducted intensive studies. At first, the situation was explained by psychological and social factors pertaining to a Ghetto lifestyle. However, it was discovered that the soils in this area contained levels of thallium so high that health department authorities never should have allowed residential development. In retrospect, the high thallium levels could be associated with the psychological problems.

In Europe, occupational thallium poisoning is covered by worker's compensation.

These previously existing contaminants (and other toxins) will likely not be limited to isolated cases. Radioactive substances and spreading landfill sites (many of which include industrial waste) will also continue to threaten our environment. The maintenance requirements of nuclear power plants are increasing faster than the risk awareness among the public. Current sanitary and protective measures associated with these industries are costly and will become even more expensive and extensive in the future.

General environmental protection measures are important not only for thallium, but for many hazardous substances. Protection measures include reducing waste (especially by recycling and, relying less on packaging) and environmental pollution (from manufacturing processes and the use of manufactured products). Batteries, for example, can now be produced without mercury. Using rechargeable batteries can reduce the total number of batteries that require mercury. Batteries will often contain lead and cadmium. Newer lithium batteries are effective and more environmentally friendly.

Biochemical Individuality and the RDA

Every organism is unique in its biochemistry. The following experiment illustrates the variance of vitamin C doses required by guinea pigs to obtain optimal benefits. Guinea pigs, like humans, cannot manufacture vitamin C on their own. The following experiment was done with several groups of guinea pigs.

The first group received 0.5 mg of vitamin C (per kg in their diet) – and 80% developed scurvy. Group 2 received 1 mg of vitamin C per kg in their diet – 25% developed scurvy. Every subsequent group received the double dose of vitamin C. In group 6 with 8 mg vitamin C there was no more scurvy, but even with another 16 mg (double the vitamin C) there were still 50% of the animals without weight gain. The ability to gain weight here is an optimal trait associated with a good/optimal state of health. You need to double the vitamin C up to 64 mg per kg to have all animals gain weight.

That means: there is a range from 0.5 mg (to prevent scurvy in the animals) to 64 mg (for all animals to gain weight). The conclusion is: **there is well over 100 times difference in the required amount of vitamin C,** and that is what biochemical individuality is all about.

Similar experiments done with students suggest a wide variance in the need for specific micronutrients. It therefore becomes important to adequately investigate every micronutrient (vitamins, minerals, etc.) to determine the optimal dose for preventing deficiency problems versus achieving optimal health.

What is called "normal" in science is 95% of the range (this applies to lab results too) of a variable. If 95% of all investigated people are 1.50 to 1.60 m tall, that range is considered "normal". However, if you live in a different country or in a different century the "normal" range varies considerably. For example, a knight's armour and bed in medieval times would be suitable today for a young teen, not an adult. This "normal" range, similar to the RDA, has many exceptions to the rule and 'one size does not fit all'.

VANADIUM

chemical symbol **V**

Normal daily requirement: ~100-300 µg?
can be poisonous in higher amounts

Functions: not well establised

Therapeutic applications: depression (including manic depression)
anorexia nervosa
cholesterol lowering
cardiac arrest
lowering blood sugar
tooth decay (strengthens teeth and bones)

Negative biological effects: none significant

Sources: fish (one serving per week is sufficient)
pepper, dill
corn

vanadium content is generally proportional
to unsaturated fat content

vanadium-rich fats include safflower,
sunflower, and olive oil.

VANADIUM

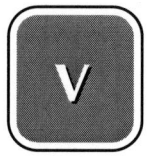

An element in the early stages of research

Until 1990, vanadium was difficult to detect and measure, especially at low concentrations. As a consequence, lab testing in recent years has often yielded contradictory results.

The daily intake of vanadium as provided by the diet is 100-300 µg on average. An adult body contains about 20-40 mg.

Ever since vanadium was used by French doctors as an all-purpose remedy during the early 1900's, its biological significance has been debated. Several reports indicate that small amounts of vanadium may be essential for life. One serving of fish per week is sufficient to cover this requirement and is the best natural source of vanadium. Other foods that have relatively high vanadium levels include buckwheat, oats, corn, black pepper, dill, safflower oil, sunflower oil, and olive oil.

Some studies have identified high vanadium levels in individuals suffering from manic depression, indicating an improvement upon following a low-vanadium diet or taking high doses of vitamin C. Excess vanadium can significantly lower lithium levels and trigger mania in which case, vitamin C and iron can be used to bring vanadium levels back down. Tranquilizers used in the treatment of bipolar depression can also lower vanadium levels.

Even though vanadium's biological target areas are unclear, the pharmacological effects of high doses have been described. In rats, enhanced insulin action was observed. In addition, comparative studies indicate that low vanadium intake in humans is associated with an increase in cardiovascular disease.

In industry, vanadium is used to produce quality steel alloys and print fabrics. Vanadium compounds are strong irritants and therefore affects mucousal tissues of the bronchi, throat, nose and eyes. In Europe, vanadium poisoning is usually covered by worker's compensation.

ZINC

chemical symbol **Zn**

recognized as an **essential** element in 1934

Normal daily requirement:

individuals over 12 years of age: 15 mg
pregnant and nursing women: 25 mg
infants up to 2, 5 and 12 months: 3, 4 and 5 mg
children up to 3, 6 and 12 years: 8, 10 and 12 mg

the therapeutic dosage is usually within the RDA

Functions:

component of over 200 enzymes in several
metabolic pathways

Therapeutic applications:

growth periods, wound healing

important for physical, mental and sexual
development of children

neurotransmitter metabolism in the brain
perception of taste and smell
skin disorders, hair loss
fertility
immune defense
protection from free radicals and radiation

hinders intestinal absorption of heavy metals
such as lead and cadmium

Negative biological effects:

prolonged elevated zinc levels decrease
copper and manganese (elements acting
antagonistically to zinc)

Sources:

meat (contains 20-50 mg/kg)
eggs (contain 5-20 mg/kg)
milk, cheese, fish, potatoes, and whole grain
products (however absorption is diminished
due to phytate constituents)

ZINC

The all-around multi-purpose essential element

An adult human contains 2-4 g of zinc. We have only slightly less zinc than iron (4-5 g in adults) in our bodies, however, many of us are still unfamiliar with zinc metabolism.

In 1869, zinc was found to be necessary for the growth of a particular mushroom, and in 1934 it was determined to be essential for animals. Carbonic anhydrase was the first zinc-containing enzyme to be isolated from red blood cells (in 1940).

Parakeratosis, a disease affecting pigs, was described in 1955. In 1963, a recurring combination of symptoms was described among children and adolescents of poorer social classes in Iran. These symptoms included general physical and mental developmental delays, testicular atrophy, anemia, liver and spleen enlargement, and skin disorders. The cause was determined to be zinc deficiency. Following zinc supplementation, symptoms were eliminated within a few months! The symptoms had been caused not only by the high phosphate and phytate levels of the Iranian diet, but by the loss of zinc due to excessive sweating in the tropical climate.

A zinc deficiency model can provide the basis for research. For example, cattle with an autosomal recessive A46 mutation have zinc deficiency due to the disruption in zinc absorption from the intestine. Their symptoms are well documented, including the effects of zinc supplementation, which has been shown to reduce immune dysfunction as a result of the deficiency (1993).

Appendix 1 describes zinc-containing enzymes and the principal functional mechanisms of trace elements. Since zinc enzymes are continually being discovered, the current total of 200 enzymes will continue to increase.

Zinc-containing enzymes are involved in:
- DNA, RNA and protein metabolism;
- growth and wound healing;
- regulation of sex hormones;
- reproductive gland function and fertility;
- membrane stabilization;
- protection from free radicals via superoxide dismutase and zinc thionine;
- inhibiting intestinal absorption of toxic heavy metals (such as lead and cadmium);

- fatty acid and prostaglandin metabolism;
- regulation of brain neurotransmitters;
- sensory functions (sight, hearing, smell, and taste);
- immune defense (cellular and humoral immunity);
- blood formation.

A milestone for zinc research occurred in 1973 when the cause of acrodermatitis enteropathica, a rare disease relatively unknown in medicine outside of pediatrics, was discovered to be a genetic disturbance of the intestinal zinc absorption mechanism. This condition, which was previously fatal in early childhood, can be treated with zinc supplementation. In the US, acrodermatitis enteropathica was also observed among patients receiving long-term parenteral (intravenous) nutrition. The cause was traced to very low zinc levels in the intravenous solutions, many of which were found to be zinc-free. These patients often experienced complete hair loss. To avoid zinc depletion during long-term intravenous treatment, it is important to monitor zinc levels frequently. Hair loss can be reversed with zinc supplementation.

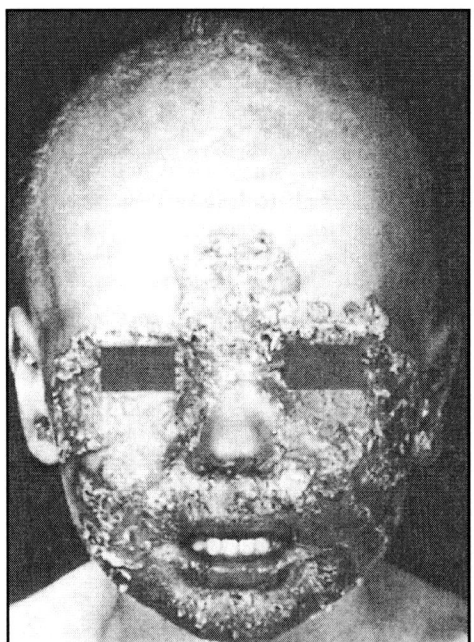 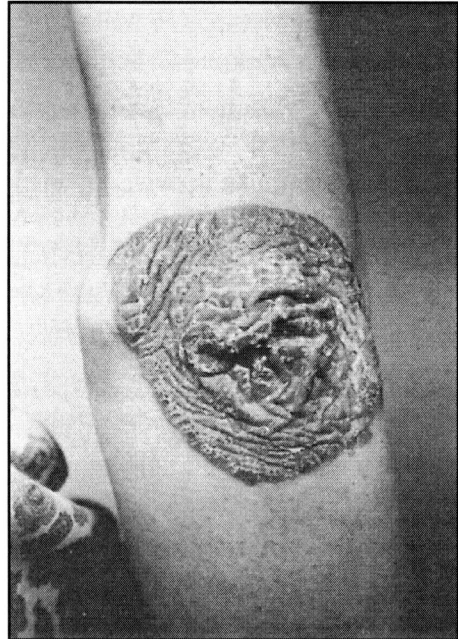

In zinc-deficient "acrodermatitis enteropathica" the skin develops lesions that look similar to those seen in psoriasis.

Zinc is required for many functions and is found practically everywhere in the human body, although concentrations differ according to location. In blood, 90% of the zinc is found within red and white blood cells and only 10% is contained in the serum (important when assessing zinc measures). In total, 60% of the body's zinc is found in skeletal muscles and 30% is found in bones. Significant concentrations are also found in the prostate, sperm and hair (useful in laboratory analysis).

Zinc content of organs (in mg/kg)

Heart 27	Kidney 37	Liver 38	Muscle 48
Bone 66	Prostate 87	Sperm 125	Hair 175

The distribution of zinc within an organ is not necessarily homogeneous. For example, in the pancreas, the majority of zinc is localized in a complex contained in the hormones insulin and glucagon inside the alpha and beta cells of the islets of Langerhans (zinc levels drop here whenever insulin excretion increases).

In cases of zinc deficiency, blood serum zinc levels drop much faster than those in erythrocytes. Serum levels rise much faster as well. Since zinc content is 10 times lower in serum than in erythrocytes, even a slight amount of hemolysis can lead to elevated serum values.

Individuals at risk for zinc deficiency include:
- pregnant and nursing women, newborns (baby formulas often contain too little zinc);
- people who have unbalanced diets ("fast food") or eat very little, such as adolescents and seniors (sometimes food in retirement homes and hospitals is less than optimal);
- people fed intravenously over prolonged periods or who frequently undergo weight loss diets;
- strict vegetarians (since high phytate levels hinder zinc absorption);
- alcoholics (due to an unbalanced diet and increased loss of zinc through the urine);
- elite athletes (due to excessive sweating and increased zinc requirements);
- those with increased zinc loss due to intestinal or skin disorders, diabetes (with increased urine loss from the kidney), infections (especially chronic), and tissue damage from surgeries, burns, heart attacks, rheumatism, collagenosis, or cancer;
- people taking D-Penicillamine (chelating agent used for rheumatism), tetracyclines, Isoniazid, Phenytoin;
- long-term users of oral contraceptives or cortisone.

Even though zinc content in food fluctuates according to soil zinc levels, there is an association between food cost and zinc content. Animal products are expensive but they are the best sources of zinc, and therefore zinc deficiency has been found frequently in people with low-income status. In Iran, for example, low-income status was associated with reduced animal product intake and, as a result, zinc deficiency symptoms.

Many diseases affect zinc metabolism. Acute and chronic infections, burns, surgery, heart attacks and cancer will lower blood zinc concentrations. This is mainly caused by an increased zinc requirement for the production of proteins (especially acute phase proteins released during stress). As an illness progresses, zinc deficiency can be worsened by reduced food intake, perspiration, wound secretion and diarrhea.

Normally, the body absorbs only 10-40% of zinc obtained from the diet. Zinc absorption is hindered by phytate, which is abundant in whole grain products. Phosphates, found in soft drinks, also decrease zinc absorption.

Since zinc is primarily found within the outer layers of a grain, zinc content falls according to the extent to which grain products are ground. Correspondingly, white flour contains the lowest amount of zinc. However, if there is sufficient time after milling (for example, when manufacturing sour dough), the phytase enzyme in the grain can dissociate various minerals, including zinc, from the phytate, thus allowing greater zinc absorption.

Zinc absorption decreases in people with albumin deficiency. Albumin is a blood protein that binds zinc (immediately following its absorption from the intestines) and transports it within the circulatory system. Excess production of gall and pancreatic fluids can also lead to zinc loss. These fluids contain elevated amounts of zinc. When they are released into the intestine, zinc is lost. During periods of zinc deficiency (and perhaps in response to high blood sugar levels) intestinal absorption is increased. Zinc is also eliminated to a certain extent through hair, perspiration and skin (especially if a skin disorder is present). Some people excrete zinc through the kidneys when intake is high. In alcoholism, pancreatic dysfunction often plays a role in the development of zinc deficiency. As a result of poor pancreatic function, alcoholics often have insufficient levels of picolinic acid which is required for optimal zinc absorption.

Elevated zinc levels in the body are rare. In some cases, elevated levels of zinc appear in the blood when zinc is mobilized from cells and tissues resulting in deficiency symptoms. By comparison, you can have a transient rise in zinc levels right after experiencing trauma or stress. High zinc intake rarely has a toxic effect since large amounts of zinc often cause intestinal irritation leading to elimination via diarrhea. Only a small amount of zinc is stored in the body's cells and tissues.

Well-intentioned, prolonged intake of higher doses of zinc (without medical supervision or laboratory feedback) is not recommended because of its antagonism with copper and manganese (and molybdenum to a lesser extent). An excess of one of these elements (zinc, copper or manganese) can unintentionally lower any of the other two equally important elements.

The lethal dose of zinc sulfate is reported to be 3-5 g and the lethal dose of zinc chloride is reported to be 6-30 g. Salt is also lethal at 30 g. Zinc overdose symptoms (especially gastric complaints, nausea, and vomiting) have been described with daily doses in excess of 100 mg when taken over a period of several weeks or months.

The following sections describe specific biochemical functions of zinc in the human body.

Zinc in childhood and puberty

Due to its role in protein synthesis and enzyme function, zinc requirements significantly increase during periods of growth. Normally we obtain larger quantities of zinc as we develop in the womb via maternal blood, in infancy via breast milk (contains more zinc than formula), and in childhood and puberty via increased food intake. Children are very sensitive to zinc deficiency. As described earlier, children in Iran and also Egypt experienced general physical, mental, and sexual developmental delays including poor growth and testicular atrophy. Zinc supplementation allowed many of these patients to regain age-related sexual development, including normal pubic hair growth and an acceleration of body growth up to 13 cm in one year. This is extremely significant for someone with halted development! During childhood, adolescence, and adulthood, zinc is important for learning, memory, concentration, and attention.

Zinc and pregnancy

Animal studies have shown that adequate maternal zinc levels are indispensable for conception and normal fetal development (especially during rapid growth in the third trimester). In one study, half of all rats fed a zinc-deficient diet from the beginning of pregnancy miscarried and the other half gave rise to birth defects. The birth defects occurred in various organs, however half involved brain abnormalities. Animals with borderline zinc deficiency had offspring with low birth weights, although none of these had a birth defect. The control group consuming an average diet with sufficient zinc levels (but without zinc supplementation) had offspring with normal birth weights and no birth defects.

In animal studies, zinc deficiency during pregnancy has also been found to weaken the immune system. This effect has been shown to carry over into three subsequent generations – a surprising phenomenon which has yet to be fully explained.

Special attention to the signs of zinc deficiency should be given to pregnant women who are diabetic, or alcoholic, as well as pregnant teens who have higher growth-related zinc requirements than adults.

Zinc deficiency plays an important role in the development of fetal alcoholic syndrome. Elevated hormone levels during pregnancy also contribute to zinc deficiency and copper excess. This excess of copper is associated with post-partum depression and autism.

Zinc and the immune system

Significant zinc deficiency often leads to a weakened immune system. This is apparent in patients with acrodermatitis enteropathica (described above), where zinc deficiency contributes to the following: a reduction in the size of lymph nodes, thymus and spleen; a decrease in T-lymphocytes and their activity against tumor cells; and the fall of immunoglobulin G levels.

In cancer clinics, zinc deficiency was repeatedly observed among patients treated with agents that retard cell activity and replication. Zinc supplementation significantly improved patients' general well-being. This included faster wound healing, less hair loss and improvements in other conditions involving skin and mucous membranes.

Zinc and athletic performance

Zinc increases muscular strength and endurance since it is required to increase muscle mass. Athletes often have a high carbohydrate diet that is relatively low in zinc. While a normal person loses about 1.5 mg of zinc daily through perspiration, this can rise up to 6 mg (four times the normal amount!) during strenuous physical activity. Similar observations have been made among heavy laborers and even those accustomed to hot working conditions.

Zinc promotes wound healing

Since antiquity, zinc ointments have been known to improve wound healing. The zinc content of skin around a wound is higher than normal. Lower leg abscesses are often chronic conditions that can last for several years. They usually occur as a result of circulatory problems in arteries and/or veins. In addition to treating the underlying problem, zinc supplementation was beneficial for patients who did not respond to conventional treatment. A controlled study involving 104 hospital patients of various ages was conducted. They received identical capsules containing either 220 mg of zinc sulfate or 220 mg of lactose (placebo). The average healing time for patients in the zinc treatment group was 32 days versus 77 days for those in the placebo group.

Wound healing can also be promoted by zinc supplementation after surgical operations or burn trauma. It has been estimated that the average daily zinc loss following surgery is approximately 30 mg (possibly up to 600 mg). In all surgical facilities (especially in burn and emergency units), this should be taken into consideration as a preventive measure to reduce complications during and after surgery.

Zinc has also been used in the treatment of skin disorders including acne, psoriasis, hair loss (especially alopecia areata), and skin changes associated with diabetes.

Zinc has proven to be important for the metabolism of cysteine, an amino acid found in skin and hair (especially in keratin). There is also a key zinc-dependent enzyme involved in the lipid synthesis of skin cells. Patients with atopic dermatitis (includes eczema) benefit from using zinc because they often have altered skin lipid composition.

Zinc and aging

Zinc deficiency is common in older people. Several factors likely contribute to this: unbalanced diet/eating habits; increased zinc requirements; and increased loss due to illness. Seniors often have an increased need for zinc but unfortunately their ability to absorb zinc is compromised.

Zinc and the brain

Research literature has reported neurological and psychiatric conditions as a result of, or in association with, zinc deficiency. Zinc concentrations differ in various regions of the brain.

One of zinc's functions as a component of various enzymes is to regulate the synthesis and degradation of neurotransmitters (especially the amino acid-based neurotransmitters glutamate and GABA). Zinc acts as a modulator for amino acid receptors, particularly NMDA receptors. Zinc can lower excitability by moderating the NMDA receptor release of the excitatory neurotransmitter glutamate – significant in strokes (CVA's) and hyper-stimulated states with convulsions (epileptic seizures).

Zinc modulates the activity of glutamate decarboxylase, which is necessary for the production of gamma aminobutyric acid (GABA). GABA is the most important inhibitory brain neurotransmitter. GABA levels are low when zinc levels are low, resulting in reduced inhibition and prevailing nerve cell stimulation.

Zinc plays a role in the storage of biogenic amines (such as histamine) in nerve cell synaptic vesicles and is involved in rapid axonal transport. Histamine, a brain neurotransmitter, regulates electrical activity in the nucleus accumbens – an area of the brain responsible for behavior responses, filtering incoming sensory information, and communicating with the hypothalamus, ventral tegmentum, and amygdala.

Decreased zinc levels have been observed in depression, psychosis, senile dementia, and mental retardation.

Zinc is a significant calcium antagonist. Calcium antagonism is an important mechanism of action for several drugs that act on the brain, promote circulation and activate metabolic functions.

It is suspected that zinc regulates the binding of encephalins at receptor sites, protecting against fatty acid peroxidation (which causes nerve cell injury).

Anorexia nervosa and chronic alcoholism are associated with diminished zinc concentrations in the brain hippocampal area. This suggests that zinc has a role in the limbic system (emotion center) and hormonal processes of the hypothalamus and hypophysis.

Alcohol-dementia and Alzheimer's disease share similar symptoms. Zinc-dependant liver enzymes are compromised in alcohol-dementia. These same enzymes are found in the brain and, when compromised, can alter brain function and cause dementia. From this we can argue that zinc deficiency has a major role in Alzheimer's disease. In classic hepatic encephalopathy, a liver disease (usually alcohol-induced) that causes dementia, compromised liver enzyme activity as a result of zinc deficiency is suspected as follows: by reduction of glutamine neurotransmitters normally destroyed by glutamate dehydrogenase; by diminished urease production as a result of diminished ornithine carbamoyl transferase; and by diminished glutamine production as a result of diminished glutamine synthetase (this causes ammonium levels to rise, which is as damaging to the brain as diminished urease production). All of these enzymes and their activities are localized within the brain, liver and muscles.

Zinc, sensory organs and vitamin A

Zinc is important for the senses of taste and smell. Disturbances in these senses are typically accompanied by zinc deficiency. These symptoms are often overlooked by medical practitioners due to their slow and subtle development. If the taste or smell disturbance is caused by zinc deficiency alone, then zinc supplementation can normalize these senses.

Vitamin A metabolism is disrupted when zinc is deficient. Zinc is required to mobilize vitamin A from the liver and transport it through the circulatory system to the retina. The retinol-binding protein required for vitamin A transport is a zinc-dependent protein produced in the liver. In the retina, zinc assists in vitamin A metabolism. The production of retinaldehyde from retinol requires alcohol dehydrogenase – a zinc-dependent enzyme. It is well known that vitamin A deficiency causes night blindness. Zinc deficiency plays an integral role in this process.

In some cases, zinc deficiency may play a role in optic nerve damage. This observation was made in patients with acrodermatitis enteropathica (mentioned above). When these patients were treated with zinc supplementation, optic nerve damage no longer occurred.

Miscellaneous information

Zinc deficiency has been observed during acute and chronic infections, acute and chronic tissue injuries, collagenosis and rheumatoid arthritis.

Mild zinc deficiency has been found in dialysis patients. In these patients, a diminished sense of taste was often the earliest sign. Zinc supplementation resulted in increased alkaline phosphatase activity (suggesting improved kidney function).

Some ENT (ear, nose, and throat) clinics recommend zinc supplementation for sensory deafness. It was discovered that the inner ear was less sensitive to sound under zinc deficiency. Zinc-based synapses were found in a group of nerve cells of the inner ear called the nucleus cochlearis. Positive results have also been reported in the treatment of age-related deafness and tinnitus (ringing in the ear).

Due to the high zinc content of seminal fluid, it seems possible that an existing or borderline zinc deficiency can be worsened by frequent sexual intercourse. More serious zinc deficiency leads to a decrease in testicular size and lower sperm counts.

Gynecologists are now reporting that zinc plays a role in female hormone levels and fertility. Several hormones (including the hypophysial gonadotropins LH and FSH that are important for women) form dissociable zinc-protein-hormone complexes through which hormonal activation takes place.

Both male and female sex organs contain large amounts of zinc. Low zinc levels are often found in women and these levels plummet further with oral contraceptive use. Low zinc levels can become more problematic when a woman is pregnant (due to vomiting) or breastfeeding. One gynecologist commented on the "fascinating idea that zinc is so closely connected to the propagation of life."

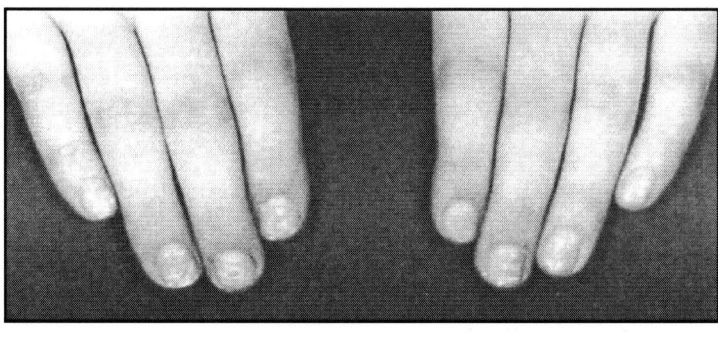

Fingernail white spots are a sign of zinc deficiency

Positive results with zinc supplementation have been found in patients with low blood pressure, cold extremities, menstrual complaints and Wilson's disease (a rare copper storage disease).

After a 1967 discovery that arthritis-like symptoms appeared in chicks with zinc deficiency, several reports on polyarthritis patients were found describing zinc supplementation reducing morning stiffness and joint swelling which enabled greater walking distances. Similar results were observed in cases of psoriatic-arthritis. To a certain extent, lab results also indicate a decline in arthritic inflammatory immunoglobulin reactions. Zinc is suspected to play a role in the following: improving blood sugar utilization in cells, resulting in better energy levels; stabilizing membranes, especially those of lysosomes; increasing cellular immunity and anti-inflammatory effects via the regulation of prostaglandin synthesis.

Prolonged zinc supplementation is often paired with copper supplementation (sometimes with a time separation) in order to prevent copper levels from dropping. The beneficial effects of zinc are enhanced when copper is present. Even so, copper supplementation is not always advised, especially when treating patients with potential copper excess problems (associated with hormonal depression, paranoia, and fatigue).

Zinc deficiency hinders insulin activity. Some substances (such as Alloxan) can form insoluble compounds with zinc which may trigger diabetes. Low zinc levels have not been found in diabetics except in those cases where arteriosclerosis is also present.

Like vitamin E, zinc stabilizes cellular membranes and protects cells from peroxidative damage. Within cells, zinc thionein and superoxide dismutase (SOD) provide important protection against free radicals.

Zinc impedes the damaging effects of cadmium, lead and mercury in part by contributing to their increased elimination.

Zinc-finger molecules (zinc containing proteins with finger-like structures) regulate the proliferation and differentiation of cells and tissues by influencing gene expression. Zinc is required for the binding of zinc-finger-containing transcription factors to DNA and for hormone-receptor interactions (especially those involving estrogen, glucocorticoids, and thyriod hormones).

Zinc and acid-base balance

Zinc deficiency influences the activity of carbonic anhydrase (CA) in the lungs, kidneys, placenta and liver. CA, a particularly well-known zinc-dependent enzyme, facilitates the following chemical reaction in a split-second:

$$CO_2 + H_2O \longleftarrow CA \longrightarrow H_2CO_3 \longleftrightarrow H^+ + HCO_3^-$$

Without CA, this reaction would take about 100 seconds to occur spontaneously. If CO_2 is removed from the equation, H_2CO_3 (carbonic acid) falls and the amount of available hydrogen (H$^+$) ions decreases. With CA, this reaction proceeds quickly and allows the body to eliminate CO_2 and to lower H+ ion concentration!

This reaction takes place during the elimination of CO_2 in the lungs. Red blood cells take only one second to flow through the smallest blood vessels in the lungs! In cases of CA deficiency, the elimination of CO_2 is diminished, leading to acid build-up within the body (respiratory acidosis). This build-up is enhanced by physical activity. The same reaction takes place during pregnancy in the placenta. Zinc deficiency makes CO_2 exchange from the fetus to the mother more difficult (in this case acidosis develops in the unborn child).

This reaction is also important in the kidneys for the elimination of H$^+$ ions. To compensate for sodium loss, one Na$^+$ ion is absorbed for every H$^+$ ion released into the urine. Zinc deficiency therefore increases sodium, potassium and magnesium loss which can lead to serious heart muscle problems.

CA is also used to form acid salts in the gastric mucosa. Zinc deficiency, and therefore CA deficiency, causes insufficient gastric acid production. Gastric acid loss is especially consequential for protein digestion. Without adequate gastric acid, many foods remain in the stomach longer, creating a full sensation or nausea. Due to insufficient acidity, residual bacteria will induce unnecessary fermentation which often leads to bloating. The resulting loss of appetite is a classic symptom of zinc deficiency. Fullness or nausea followed by bloating and a loss of appetite can continue in a cyclical pattern if you are zinc-deficient. In these cases, if you avoid protein – which is rich in zinc – to prevent digestive problems, then you are at risk of further depleting zinc.

Since CA is also utilized in the urease cycle (urea and ammonia removal) in the liver, zinc deficiency can contribute to elevated ammonia concentrations which are damaging to the brain (hepatic encephalopathy). Zinc supplementation in this case results in improved metabolism and psychological brain function.

Lab zinc values

Other than hair mineral analysis (and the examples given in the lab chapter), two additional lab tests are particularly important when measuring this trace element. One test involves monitoring alkaline phosphatase (a zinc-dependent enzyme) levels before and after zinc supplementation. An increase of these levels after zinc administration indicates possible zinc deficiency. Another sensitive method involves the determination of serum binding capacity for zinc. Binding capacity rises with zinc deficiency.

METALLOTHIONEIN, ZINC, AND HEAVY METALS

Zinc and metallothionein (MT) are intimately involved in metal regulation. Toxic mercury, for example, can bind inside the "s" configuration of MT where it would no longer be free to do harm. MT can bind up to 13 ions of copper providing a regulatory mechanism to balance zinc and copper levels. MT has the greatest affinity for mercury followed by copper, cadmium, silver, and zinc. Glutathione disulphide helps to release and exchange zinc for other metal ions. MT is found in high concentrations where heavy metals are detoxified - in the kidney, liver, and intestines.

The 'signal' to manufacture/induce the thionein component is provided by zinc, copper, cadmium, mercury, bismuth, gold, and other non-metallic compounds. Reduced glutathione found predominantly in the liver, kidney, spleen, and pancreas, helps to load zinc into thionein so it can be 'preloaded' with zinc to form active MT. Emotional stress, injury, and nuclear radiation can also induce the manufacture of MT. MT proteins are found in all cells and help us to protect from toxic metals circulating in the blood.

MT is also found in brain tissue as a factor that inhibits neuronal growth. MT has a role in brain cell pruning important in the nerve cell development and connectivity. If MT proteins are compromised, especially during development, it would be difficult to maintain optimal neurotransmitter levels. MT also has a role in behavior as the amygdala (the socialization and emotional memory area) and the hippocampus (involved in memory, learning, and behavior) have high concentrations of MT.

MT is found in the intestines, pancreas, and epithelial cells of the upper digestive tract and skin. MT prevents intestinal yeast overgrowth and intestinal inflammation. When MT binds to toxic metals in the intestinal lining it prevents them from entering the bloodstream. MT allows optimal zinc availability in the intestine to help breakdown casein and gluten. MT is important for the immune system, is involved in stomach acid manufacture, and plays a role in the discrimination of taste.

Zinc, selenium, glutathione, vitamin A and cysteine are important nutrients to promote MT formation and function.

Section

2

CLINICAL
APPLICATIONS

CLINICAL APPLICATIONS

Testing for trace minerals: body fluid versus tissue measures

Over the past 20-25 years, medical laboratory tests for trace elements have undergone remarkable improvements in resolution and quality. Much of today's knowledge has resulted from their enhancement. Samples for trace mineral testing are usually obtained from body fluids (typically blood serum or urine) or tissues (including organs, red blood cells, or hair). Blood tests that use the 'fluid' portion of blood (serum or plasma) are considered body fluid measures, not tissue measures. Blood tests that use the red blood cell portion of blood are considered tissue measures.

Obtaining tissue samples from organs can be an invasive procedure for the patient, whereas hair samples are much easier to collect. Hair has been used formally in forensic medicine but only recently as an assessment tool for patient treatment.

Blood tests are commonly used for investigation because measurements of highly concentrated elements (especially calcium, magnesium, potassium and iron) can readily be made.

Routine blood tests (excluding red blood cell measures) have two predominant disadvantages. Due to the high water content of blood, many trace elements are diluted beyond the limit of detection ("watered-down"). Much like blood sugar values, which are influenced by sugar intake, trace element blood values fluctuate when patients take a meal with the trace element before sample collection.

The trace element content of food and intestinal absorption rates will vary greatly from person to person. If you have an empty stomach at the time of sample collection or, if you have consumed a meal rich in trace elements just before sample collection, then your blood values will vary considerably.

Fluctuating blood values of calcium and magnesium are especially worth noting here. Blood values for calcium can only be deemed useful if measured 48 hours after commencing a calcium, magnesium and phosphate balanced diet. Due to the substantial effort required to carry out this diet, it seems impractical (see also Magnesium chapter). Long-term calcium deficiency leads to osteoporosis at a later age. Since normal calcium levels are usually found in blood tests of patients with this condition, these measurements are unsuitable for the diagnosis or prevention of osteoporosis.

For years, magnesium supplements have been advertised in medical journals advising that "warning symptoms occur before serum levels drop." This is accurate because a magnesium deficiency can occur when blood serum values are within normal range. In these cases, magnesium supplementation should begin when deficiency symptoms are evident. Magnesium deficiency can be confirmed in these cases when symptoms improve. This is considered a "diagnosis by treatment." It is questionable whether it is worth investing the time and money on magnesium blood testing when a trial with magnesium supplements can simultaneously diagnose and treat the patient.

Fluctuating blood values (excluding red blood cell measures) of lithium, copper (in the context of rheumatism), and lead have been described in their respective chapters. Fluctuating blood values of zinc and iron are also worth noting. Both zinc and iron blood measures vary greatly when red blood cells in the sample break open (hemolysis) during improper collection (a common occurrence). Circadian and daily fluctuations of zinc and iron also vary significantly. The blood measure of either of these elements will be high unless tests are performed by waiting until sufficient time has passed after dosing. When iron levels are low, serum ferritin measures are useful to confirm iron deficiency.

While the human body contains substantial amounts of calcium, it holds only 10-30 mg of the trace elements iodine, selenium and molybdenum. Even with today's advanced technologies, these minute quantities easily approach their limit of detection. Additional problems arise when lab chemicals and the materials used for blood draws (needles, syringes, glass draw tubes, etc.) contain small amounts of the material to be tested. This contamination risk threatens the accuracy of results and applies particularly to blood analyses involving aluminum, chromium, cobalt, manganese, vanadium, and zinc. Hair is an excellent test material because you can measure more elements than in either blood or urine tests alone. Hair retains trace elements (deposited over a two to three month period) thus allowing levels to accumulate such that they can be measured. In some cases, blood and urine tests can complement hair mineral analysis. Supplemental blood tests can sometimes verify hair measures. Hidden copper toxicity seen by hair mineral analysis is not uncommon and blood measures may or may not confirm this finding. In some cases of heavy metal (especially mercury) toxicity, blood or hair analysis values appear normal. Abnormal levels are more likely to appear when mobilized by urine challenge protocols.

The limitations of lab test values can be seen by examining home tap water samples obtained at different times of the day. Mildly elevated copper levels were observed in one home's tap water. The water also contained 481 ppm of calcium (hard water). The home owner installed a decalcifier. Decalcifiers are water softeners that exchange calcium in the water for sodium and often add phosphate and silicate to reduce acidity. Copper levels increased after decalcification despite adding more silicate to the decalcifier. Water samples were taken from various taps at different times and the following results were obtained:

Water before decalcification: 0.08 mg Cu/L (in comparison, water from a neighboring town had 0.05 mg Cu/L)

Water after decalcification: 0.24 mg Cu/L (at noon, kitchen)
0.36 mg Cu/L (at noon, guest washroom)
1.12 mg Cu/L (first sample of the day, kitchen)

While normal copper levels were found before decalcification and, otherwise, only moderately higher measurements were detected during the day, a 14-fold increase in copper concentration was discovered in the first sample of the day after the water had been standing in the pipes overnight. This should be taken into consideration when washing hair, and more importantly for health reasons, when preparing morning coffee.

These findings indicate that even common laboratory tests can have problems or limitations, and that their interpretation should be based on sound medical knowledge. A preferable solution is trace element analysis of hair, although it is definitely not ideal for every situation and does not render other methods superfluous. There have been enormous improvements in this field in the past few years, partly due to the merger of at least two investigation techniques (in particular ICP and MS). Since hair analysis is also offered by laboratories that may operate with outdated equipment, lack quality control standards, or employ unqualified personnel, the medical community often doubts its validity. Unfortunately, some hairdressers offer hair analysis (but only test mechanical qualities such as elasticity) and subsequently recommend expensive products containing vitamins and trace elements. For this reason, hair analysis should probably more precisely be referred to as hair mineral analysis. Scientifically, for some fields this technique has been undisputed for years – for example, in diagnosing an unclear recent death – in forensic investigations, especially in the diagnoses of arsenic or mercury poisoning. Hair samples from the past can also be analyzed (e.g. the hair from Napoleon, Beethoven, or ancient mummies).

ICP and MS are the most commonly used techniques for hair mineral analysis. ICP stands for Inductive Coupled high frequency Plasma emission spectrometry. This method has been recognized for a long time. The material to be tested is heated to such extremes (several thousand degrees Celsius) that it is converted to its plasma state. Its atoms then emit light at specific wavelengths characteristic of each element. MS signifies Mass Spectroscopy. At very high temperatures, the test material becomes a stream of electrically charged particles that are deflected by a magnetic field and strike a detector. The degree of deflection is proportional to the size of the charge and inversely proportional to the atomic mass of the particle. Each substance produces a characteristic pattern that can be identified. Reliability and accuracy is improved by automatically correcting values for isobaric conditions.

In the last few years, it has become possible to combine the two technically distinct methods ICP and MS in one apparatus. As a result, multiple elements can be analyzed simultaneously within a large measurement range and with great accuracy. The high degree of sensitivity allows for elements to be analyzed at concentrations barely detectable by other (and more laborious) methods. Over 60 elements are traceable below 0.1 ng/mL (or ppb), and therefore only very small test quantities are required. The detectors enable analyses over a wider concentration range up to 200 ppm. A reliable identification of all elements present in a sample is made possible by duplicate measurements and, especially with ICP-MS, the complementation of values derived from every isotope of a particular element.

This technology has offered medical, biological and other research fields the possibility of using non-radioactive, stable isotopes for trace element testing. However, the technical effort required to carry out this technique is so considerable that it is not feasible in a regular lab. A high level of knowledge is necessary to apply this technology, and therefore a scientist such as a physicist or chemist with thorough practical experience with these techniques is required.

More simplified techniques can be used to measure many trace elements and abnormalities such as lead and arsenic poisoning without much difficulty. For elements such as zinc, selenium, chromium and molybdenum, the most common and medically significant problem is insufficient intake. When these elements are present at very low levels, older measurement methods begin to approach their physical and technical limits. Furthermore, many laboratories fail to indicate which measurement technique they use and its respective measurement range, making it difficult to standardize results. Some elements such as vanadium were difficult for high-tech labs to measure until about 1990.

The longer you are engaged with trace minerals and their medical consequences, the more you can appreciate the possibility of studying several elements simultaneously. A multiple element analysis is primarily done for several reasons. Before investigating, problematic trace elements may not be known. More often, problems are found for several trace elements as opposed to just one (examples of this will follow). This is generally referred to as a multiple deficiency syndrome. Also, it is often interesting to determine the values for elements that act as antagonists of those found at abnormal levels. It is less expensive to do a multiple element hair analysis than several single element analyses.

Hair root cells, like other cells in the body, take up nutrients and trace elements from the bloodstream. This occurs by passive transport (according to concentration gradients) as well as by active transport. Exchange events known to occur in the blood also take place in other tissues and influence their composition. Therefore, values measured from hair should not simply be interpreted as an "extension" of blood values. Some heavy metals are deposited more readily in certain areas of the body than in hair. For example, the liver contains arsenic deposits; lead accumulates in bone; and mercury builds up in the nervous system. Just as for blood tests, not all hair analyses are alike. Hair differs not only in color but also with respect to its chemical structure, particularly the number of sulfur and amino groups present. These groups each have distinctive binding capacities and affinities for various trace elements.

One experiment traced zinc-65 in hair only two hours after its uptake. It is unlikely that the element could pass from the bloodstream to the hair root sheath cells by passive transport in two hours. That being said, within two hours zinc may be able to enter the hair-root; it is not likely that it could, in such a short time, make its way into the dead part of the hair outside of the scalp where the hair sample is taken from. It is unclear whether zinc is secreted by the sweat glands and enters hair from the outside.

Hair analysis should be sensibly classified and interpreted with medical knowledge, just like other commonly used assessment tools: blood, urine, and spinal fluid testing, imaging (e.g. X-ray studies) and other medical findings. Even among patients with serious rheumatism, 20% fail to have the typical rheumatism-factor in their blood. Similarly, an inconspicuous X-ray or CT scan would not rule out the presence of headaches. This reasoning should be kept in mind when considering hair analysis, which is much less expensive and provides an analysis of 30 trace elements.

In summary, hair is especially suited for trace element investigations because it grows slowly, incorporating elements from the body and blood by uptake through hair root cells. In comparison to rapid uptakes observed in blood tests, hair analysis provides an average value corresponding to the last 2-4 months (depending on hair length and individual differences in growth rate). This average value over a longer period of time makes hair analysis especially informative for many medical inquiries. Daily fluctuations are not as important as long-term intake, since a single day of insufficient intake of a particular element such as iron would not immediately develop into a medical problem such as anemia.

Hair analysis is also advantageous because samples are easily obtainable. The 1-2 g of hair used for the analysis does not require preservation or extra preparation, nor is it sensitive to external influences (except for direct contamination). The hair is cut close to the scalp at the nape (without roots) and should not be longer than 4-5 cm per strand. Hair at the end of a long ponytail could be several years old and would give outdated results as well as increase the risk of contamination. The hair does not need to be washed since it is cleaned with special solutions in the lab. If possible, it should not be color treated, bleached or permed. If insufficient head hair is available, samples can be taken from other areas of the body as long as they have had minimal exposure to sweat or other contaminants.

Comparative hair measures should only be made between hair samples from the same local body area. Hair from the head and pubic hair have different properties and growth rates and will therefore provide different results.

Meanwhile, it is also possible to determine average values for trace elements by monitoring red blood cells, which have a lifespan of approximately 120 days. However this analysis method is not available for all trace elements and standard deviations have not been well established (versus conventional blood tests). Red blood cell testing is also currently much more expensive than hair analysis. With time, red blood cell measures may become available as routine laboratory tests.

The result of an ICP-MS hair analysis, costing $80-120 USD depending on how many elements are measured (and the amount of additional elaborations), can resemble the following three patient examples shown on pages 141 to 147.

CLINICAL ASSESSMENT

This section outlines the therapeutic application of trace element research

A pregnant woman takes "iron for the blood" and "calcium for the bones", yet few people know that according to modern medical recommendations, she should also take extra zinc. In veterinary medicine, grazing animals are given trace elements in the form of a salt lick when soil analyses reveal deficiencies. Trace elements are used intensively in the training programs of elite athletes. To combat dehydration in desert and tropical environments, the United States Army recently developed a rehydration beverage containing optimal doses of magnesium not found in most sports drinks.

As these examples illustrate, there are various reasons for considering the use of trace elements:

1. **A trace element is deficient or missing,** such as in iron deficiency anemia. The intake of this element represents the optimal and complete treatment of the disease. A simple case such as this is rather rare in medicine.

2. **During periods of elevated requirement,** additional intake of trace elements may be necessary. Often there is no precipitating illness (or not yet). In addition to pregnancy, increased requirements can develop as a result of illness (such as an increased zinc requirement due to surgery or burns). This applies to conditions that hinder the intestinal absorption of trace elements or contribute to their increased loss through the intestinal tract or urine.

   An increased requirement exists to a certain extent in children, seniors, the sick, and those who have an unbalanced diet (and often in people who over-eat and consume excess calories). The requirements are also rising in industrialized countries where, due to factors in agriculture and food-processing, the diet does not contain every trace element and vitamin in sufficient quantity.

3. **Diseases with several causes and influencing factors.** An increasing number of illnesses are being identified to have many possible causes. Between different people and different diseases, individual factors can play varying roles. In this sense, trace element problems can contribute to the worsening of existing diseases or can partially cause an illness directly. Accordingly, trace elements are being used to an increasing degree as supplementary treatment for cancer patients. The beneficial

effects of trace elements can be optimized by supporting the treatment with laboratory data that indicate which elements are low.

However, laboratory results cannot usually predict the outcome of trace element supplementation, except for when a trace element deficiency is the only or most important factor contributing to an illness. A supplementation program is worth trying when previous treatment has been unsatisfactory. After some time, laboratory analysis shows the success of trace element supplementation, after which further decisions are made about how to proceed. This concept is generally used in other areas of medicine as well.

4. **Free radical considerations**

Free radicals are highly reactive compounds. They are generated during various metabolic stages (where the body often has protective mechanisms in place) and are required to a certain degree for normal metabolic functions. Free radicals play a role in biological events such as inflammation, infection, immunity and cancer development. They can be released in high amounts by chemicals, energetic/radioactive rays and metabolic disturbances, leading to negative biological effects.

Free radical mechanisms are now considered important factors in an increasing number of diseases, especially those classified as "diseases of civilization", degenerative, age-related or chronic.

The following compounds (commonly known as **free radical scavengers** or **antioxidants**) are found in body cells as protective agents against free radicals:

- Glutathione peroxidase (GSH) – every molecule contains four selenium atoms
- Superoxide dismutase (SOD) – there are several forms containing manganese, zinc or copper
- Vitamin C (water soluble), vitamin E (fat soluble), beta carotene, and CoQ10

These antioxidants are not found in equal quantities within all cells. Metabolically active cells contain increased amounts. In addition, these compounds are not dispersed evenly throughout the whole cell. Optimal protection does not occur through one factor alone (even if it is available in large amounts), but through the collective availability and interaction of all factors (the "antioxidant orchestra").

5. **Toxic heavy metals** (most commonly by lead, cadmium and mercury) can be counteracted by the intake of antagonistic trace elements or substances that promote the elimination of heavy metals. For example, in

Wilson's disease (see Copper chapter), life-threatening copper levels can be reduced by the antagonist zinc. Obviously, heavy metal intoxication should be prevented whenever possible. Other metals found in excess include aluminum, iron (hemochromatosis), and silver.

Trace element applications can be classified as follows:

One trace element is deficient or missing

Magnesium is a good example. Some marketing strategies have tried to ascribe the reputation of a universal remedy. This overstatement is as incorrect as the opposite belief that magnesium is ineffective and unimportant. The cost of trace element prescriptions is covered only if a deficiency has been officially proven. This applies to magnesium, although deficiency symptoms may appear well before blood values fall outside of the normal range. This phenomenon was described in the laboratory chapter as "symptoms appearing before serum levels indicate an abnormality." With magnesium, a blood test is almost more expensive than a prescription (which would be used as a trial treatment); if magnesium supplementation alleviates the symptoms, the suspected diagnosis is confirmed (also known as an *ex juvantibus* diagnosis). Otherwise, the results would have to be explained by a placebo effect (or coincidence).

More than one trace element is deficient

Costs are only covered by the health care system in some cases. Pregnant women are given "iron for the blood" and "calcium for the bones." Some of these preparations also contain additional ingredients such as zinc, folic acid and other micronutrients.

Aside from some supplements for patients on kidney dialysis, some health insurance plans also cover similar supplements for cancer patients.

The disadvantage of store-bought multi-supplements is that ingredients are present in fixed, predetermined amounts. Some pregnant women, for example, may need more iron or less calcium than is present in a given supplement. If only two elements are deficient then they can easily be taken separately. However it is expensive and difficult to follow a treatment plan if several elements are required.

Several trace elements are deficient

As shown by the hair mineral analysis examples in the following section and by research and patient results, the occurrence of multiple trace element deficiencies in one person is common. This is referred to as multiple deficiency syndrome. Often this is also associated with mild heavy metal

2 to 3 mg. copper . . . . . 15mg. zinc

intoxication (usually due to environmental pollution). Heavy metals exhibit their damaging effects often by displacing other elements such as zinc or selenium from their sites of action in the body. The elimination of heavy metals can be accelerated by taking a corresponding chemical or biochemical antagonist element. For example, selenium promotes mercury excretion. Consuming fish that contain an increased amount of mercury is not as risky as lead intoxication from other sources since fish also contain a relatively high amount of selenium. Different trace elements and certain supplements promote the elimination of various toxic heavy metals.

There is no "universal antidote supplement" for all toxic heavy metals. On the other hand, antagonism also occurs between essential trace elements like copper and zinc. If one takes increased amounts of zinc over a prolonged period of time, his/her copper levels will decrease. The lower the copper levels were to begin with, the more likely copper deficiency problems are to develop. Zinc has been described as an important trace element, therefore deficiencies should be addressed. However, taking in excessive amounts over a longer period of time (according to the belief that "more is better") would not have a greater benefit and could even promote copper deficiency. Copper can be fatal, in which case there is often an underlying zinc deficiency. (This has happened not only to native people in the US but also to infants in southern Germany.) Some trace element supplements, even if taken in recommended quantities, already contain a high amount of copper *15 mg zinc* in relation to zinc (2-3 mg of copper, which is within the daily requirement range, compared to only a fraction of the 15 mg zinc requirement). Long-term intake of supplements at an incorrect zinc-to-copper ratio can lead to elevated copper and deficient zinc (and manganese and molybdenum) levels.

Even though intentions may be good, an unnecessarily high intake of trace element supplements can create undesirable effects in the long run. Before increasing the dosage of any trace element supplement, a diagnosis should be determined by laboratory analysis. This also applies to long-term intake of combination supplements if their individual components fall at or over the daily requirement range. Laboratory evaluations should be performed more frequently if the dosages exceed daily requirements.

Since the body has a limited capacity to absorb most elements and cannot adjust suddenly to deficiencies, taking high doses of trace elements within a short period of time is not recommended. Dosages should be determined on a case-by-case basis following a laboratory diagnosis. Everyone understands that taking a complete package of 100 tablets all at once for iron deficiency would be absurd (this would also cause side effects such as intestinal discomfort). It is recommended to take most supplements on a daily basis (1-3 tablets) over an extended time period. On the other hand, insufficient dosages, such as a very low daily intake or taking only one tablet per week, would fail to result in any improvement or would at least delay improvement.

Taking individual doses of several trace elements and vitamins on a daily basis over a long time period would be difficult, whether they are taken separately or as combination supplements. The following method, made possible by specialized compounding facilities, could be helpful.

The medical practitioner can prescribe a mixture of various components (thus formulating a mixture with quality ingredients and optimal doses). This combination can then be put together by a specialized compounding facility that is familiar with these prescriptions and has experience formulating them. The medical practitioner and the compounder need to remember that the individual components should not interfere with each other in terms of intestinal absorption or body storage. This can be achieved by using trace elements in the chelated form (relatively more expensive) and specialized yeasts (such as dried, selenium yeast instead of selenium salts). Chelation often occurs in the body to facilitate absorption. For example, zinc is absorbed more easily when bound to picolinate, and the low absorption of vitamin B12 can be enhanced by the intrinsic factor. The following section provides an example describing this principle in more detail.

A combination of several trace elements and vitamins

Here we will refer to the hair mineral analysis example of a 54 year old woman with knee arthrosis (Case 1) on page 141.

For many patients, daily dosages of trace elements and/or vitamins can be gradually lowered over an extended period of time. Ultimately, the length and intensity of a supplementation program is an individual decision (often also in consideration of cost). If the full dosage is not taken every day, the prescribed quantity of capsules will last for a longer period of time.

Prescribed supplements are not intended to replace good nutrition

The rate and degree of intestinal absorption, losses through urine, stool, perspiration and menstruation, as well as metabolic requirements of individual micronutrients are not identical in all people. This range of biological differences means that everyone has individual metabolic and trace element requirements.

There are different recommendations in different countries regarding trace minerals, vitamins and other micronutrients. For example, the vitamin C deficiency disease scurvy was a threat to the sailors for many centuries and killed more men than all the sea battles that fill our history books. In Germany, 60 mg of vitamin C was considered adequate for the prevention of scurvy; therefore the recommended daily allowance (RDA) was 60 mg. However, the World Health Organization (WHO) uses the value of 200 mg for this purpose and adds another 50 mg for smokers. Germany further raised the 60 mg to only 75 mg, and allows vitamin C supplements and other supplements only if they contain three times the RDA (3 x 75 = 215 mg) at maximum. If a supplier recommends taking 1-3 doses of a multi-supplement that contains 100 mg of vitamin C, the food and drug control will conclude that a person could take 300 mg in a day. Because this exceeds the permitted (3 x 75 =) 215 mg, the issuing company will have to discontinue the product and advise the consumption of only 1-2 supplements a day (so that the maximum is 2 x 100 = 200 mg). Every dose exceeding the RDA is only allowed following the same time and money-consuming efforts that every new chemical compound must undergo before it is allowed to be sold as a new pharmaceutical agent. This "three times the RDA-rule" is an example of official regulations for minerals and vitamins – these rules and limitations are different in many countries.

The dose that prevents a deficiency disease is not identical to the dose for optimal support of the body's individual biochemistry and needs. How much vitamin C do you take, for example, for the flu (and perhaps together with aspirin)? Three doses of 1 g or more? Do you consider that more than 215 mg might be a danger to your life? There are other risks that government should care more about. By law it is easier to get dangerous chemicals than the optimum trace mineral and vitamin doses for your individual biochemistry.

As medical practitioners, we want to prescribe optimum quantities for a patient to meet his/her personal requirements. With clinical experience, medical practitioners begin to recognize many problems and side effects associated with regular medications. However, micronutrients are associated with far less risk because the body knows how to handle these substances. This book aims to help achieve the optimum benefit of micronutrients.

Two-time Nobel prize winner Linus Pauling took 16-18 g of vitamin C daily over many decades and lived over 93 years with good physical and mental capacities.

The body absorbs some modern forms of trace elements better. In the case of iron, modern forms are better tolerated than the approved "ancient chemicals" (such as iron chloride). However, these newer forms are often banned for use in food products since they were unknown or overlooked at the time (often 30 or 40 years ago) when food product guidelines were developed. In Europe, in a matter laughed at by the public and the press, tonnes of cucumber that did not meet the specified requirements for geometric shape and could not be sold and therefore ended up in the garbage. The farmer was only allowed to eat it himself.

Athletes (as well as other healthy individuals) can increase their mental and physical capabilities through prophylaxis. When a previously unknown African soccer team was winning against highly ranked countries in the 1990 World Cup, the media attributed the results to particular methods employed by this team's coach. He was a nutrition specialist! In the US, nutrition consultants have been involved with Olympic teams for years. One of them wrote a book about this field called *The Doctor's Vitamin and Mineral Encyclopedia* (Hendler, 1990). Not only is it backed by proven research, it is also comprehensible to laypersons.

An educated farmer would probably smile and realize at this point that he has been practicing trace element supplementation for years, enhancing the health and vitality of his animals by providing them with salt licks corresponding to trace element deficiencies discovered in his soil. People who have walked around farm areas (at least in Europe) would certainly recognize these blocks, each having a different color according to the element it contains.

Hair mineral analysis is also used as a screening (and preventive) measure to determine heavy metal intoxications and trace element deficiencies among healthy (or still healthy) individuals. Certain laboratory deviations would prompt a recommendation to take trace element or vitamin supplements, even if disease symptoms have not yet developed. This type of supplementation is termed preventative medicine (prophylaxis) versus therapy.

Case 1 (patient number 502):
54 years old, female (P.I.)

This patient had osteoarthritis of the knee that, despite treatment, had become so painful over the years (x-ray results showed significant degenerative changes) that she could no longer play tennis (her regular sport). Her daily activities were significantly compromised. Upon consideration of knee replacement surgery, the orthopedic surgeon and the patient were deterred by the best case scenario of an artificial knee lasting only 15 years (she would then be in her late sixties). Replacement after that would be uncertain. The surgeon was reserved about recommending surgery, yet did not see any other option considering her long unsuccessful treatment history. By chance, he had heard about trace element therapy and asked one of the authors to conduct a trace element analysis with the goal of developing an appropriate supplement program.

The hair mineral analysis indicates only mild deficiencies among four trace elements: calcium, zinc, molybdenum probably (or low normal reading) and selenium. There were no significant problems with the toxic elements. The selenium value was less than 0.24 ppm and the laboratory could only accurately measure up to 0.24 ppm, given the quantity of hair and other test parameters. Therefore selenium could be 0.23 ppm at most, or substantially lower.

These results (which were not particularly grave or alarming) were combined with vitamin aspects. Also taken into consideration was that severe osteoarthritis would produce an increased amount of free radicals, potentially worsening the illness by perpetuating the condition. The patient received the following prescription:

6 capsules, to be taken in 3 divided doses during the day, containing:
Vitamin A 4000 IU; Vitamin E 100 IU; Beta carotene 15 mg;
Vitamin B1 50 mg; B2 50 mg; B5 80 mg; B6 100 mg;
Vitamin B12 50 µg; Biotin 50 µg; Folic acid 1 mg; PABA 80 mg;
Choline 20 mg; Niacinamide 300 mg;
Zinc (chelated) 10 mg; Manganese (chelated) 1 mg;
Selenium 300 µg (yeast); Chromium 25 µg (as yeast); Molybdenum 10 µg;
Magnesium 60 mg; Vitamin C (in calcium ascorbate form) 2 g.

A 75 day supply of capsules was made with the above mixture. The vitamin C in the above prescription acts as an antioxidant and increases the intestinal absorption of various trace elements (especially iron). For this reason, additional iron was left out of the prescription.

Patient number 502:
Hair mineral analysis

* calcium greater than 2000 ppm and magnesium greater than 200 ppm indicates deficiency status with mobilization of these minerals out of storage (especially from bone)
** ppm = parts per million

Mineral	Reference (ppm)			Test value	Range: Low	Normal	High
Calcium*	350	-	1650	3424		xxxxxxxx	____
Magnesium*	26	-	190	134		xxxxxxxx	
Phosphorous	135	-	275	160		xxxxxxxx	
Zinc	190	-	280	167	____	xxxxxxxx	
Silica	8	-	22	9.6		xxxxxxxx	
Chromium	0.2	-	0.6	0.49		xxxxxxxx	
Manganese	0.3	-	1.4	0.68		xxxxxxxx	
Molybdenum	0.1	-	1.3	< 0.10	____	xxxxxxxx	
Copper	8	-	48	13.3		xxxxxxxx	
Iron	11	-	24	10.1	____	xxxxxxxx	
Selenium	0.2	-	0.9	< 0.24	____	xxxxxxxx	
Cobalt	0.1	-	0.3	0.22		xxxxxxxx	
Boron	0	-	3.5	2.00		xxxxxxxx	
Gold	0.2	-	0.5	0.68		xxxxxxxx	
Silver	0.1	-	0.6	0.63		xxxxxxxx	
Platinum	0.2	-	0.5	< 0.29		xxxxxxxx	
Strontium	0.5	-	10	8.84		xxxxxxxx	
Barium	0.4	-	6	3.13		xxxxxxxx	
Vanadium	0.1	-	0.3	0.34		xxxxxxxx	
Nickel	0.2	-	1.0	0.76		xxxxxxxx	
Germanium	0.2	-	0.4	< 0.32		xxxxxxxx	
Iodine	0	-	22	< 7.3		xxxxxxxx	
Sulfur	31000	-	47000	37062		xxxxxxxx	

Toxic Minerals	Reference range			Test value	Normal	Toxic
Cadmium	0	-	0.4	< 0.05	xxxxxxx	
Lead	0	-	2.5	< 0.7	xxxxxxx	
Aluminum	0	-	5.0	5.1	xxxxxxx _	
Mercury	0	-	1.5	1.42	xxxxxxx	
Arsenic	0	-	2.0	< 1.0	xxxxxxx	

Important laboratory results are in **bold.**
In a comprehensive analysis such as this one, not all minute deviations are significant.

At the compounding facility, the daily dosage of this prescription was fit into six identical capsules ("size 0", each with a volume of 0.68 ml – about the size of a regular Aspirin tablet). The cost for the 75 day treatment came to about $275 USD. In less than three months, the patient renewed the prescription and reported that almost all of her symptoms had disappeared and that she was back playing tennis! She hoped to manage a few more years this way without knee replacement surgery and referred some of her neighbors and friends for analysis, despite living 200 km away. After one year she reported that she had experimentally reduced her daily intake, which caused her symptoms to reappear. This prompted her to resume taking the full dosage, which again led to the disappearance of her symptoms. Her treatment has now been successful for more than 15 years! The prescription can be altered at each renewal when there are changes to laboratory results or new clinical presentations.

It is common in hair mineral analysis to find numerous but small deviations. Greater deviations from the normal ranges are more rare. As this patient's case shows, the therapeutic application of trace elements can have remarkable results even when deviations are small.

Case 2 (patient number 1208)
53 year old female (G.I.): Hair mineral analysis

* calcium greater than 2000 ppm and magnesium greater than 200 ppm indicates deficiency status with mobilization of these minerals out of storage (especially from bone)
** ppm = parts per million

Mineral	Reference (ppm)			Test value	Range: Low	Normal	High
Calcium*	350	-	1650	2220		xxxxxxxx	—
Magnesium*	26	-	190	64		xxxxxxxx	
Phosphorous	135	-	275	172		xxxxxxxx	
Zinc	190	-	280	223		xxxxxxxx	
Silica	8	-	22	14.5		xxxxxxxx	
Chromium	0.2	-	0.6	0.07	____	xxxxxxxx	
Manganese	0.3	-	1.4	0.34		xxxxxxxx	
Molybdenum	0.1	-	1.3	< 0.09	—	xxxxxxxx	
Copper	8	-	48	128.6		xxxxxxxx	____
Iron	11	-	24	8.6	—	xxxxxxxx	
Selenium	0.2	-	0.9	0.37		xxxxxxxx	
Cobalt	0.1	-	0.3	< 0.15		xxxxxxxx	
Boron	0	-	3.5	0.34		xxxxxxxx	
Gold	0.2	-	0.5	< 0.80		xxxxxxxx	
Silver	0.1	-	0.6	1.12		xxxxxxxx	—
Platinum	0.2	-	0.5	0.62		xxxxxxxx	—
Strontium	0.5	-	10	5.79		xxxxxxxx	
Barium	0.4	-	6	1.76		xxxxxxxx	
Vanadium	0.1	-	0.3	0.15		xxxxxxxx	
Nickel	0.2	-	1.0	0.25		xxxxxxxx	
Germanium	0.2	-	0.4	< 0.28		xxxxxxxx	
Iodine	0	-	22	< 0.215		xxxxxxxx	
Sulfur	31000	-	47000	42072		xxxxxxxx	

Toxic Minerals	Reference range			Test value	Normal	Toxic
Cadmium	0	-	0.6	< 0.05	xxxxxxx	
Lead	0	-	3.5	10.5	xxxxxxx	_____
Aluminum	0	-	5.0	6.4	xxxxxxx	____
Mercury	0	-	2.5	0.56	xxxxxxx	
Arsenic	0	-	3.0	< 0.9	xxxxxxx	
Thallium	0	-	0.04	0.067	xxxxxxx	____
Antimony	0	-	0.06	0.043	xxxxxxx	
Beryllium	0	-	0.25	< 0.108	xxxxxxx	

Important laboratory results are in **bold**.
In a comprehensive analysis such as this one, not all minute deviations are significant.

This patient's main complaints were extreme fatigue and difficulties in concentration. In addition, she often experienced problems associated with her spine and muscles. In the year before this analysis, she had suffered from a case of bronchitis and early pneumonia for several months. She also noticed that she felt much better on her frequent business trips and that within a few days of returning home the fatigue would resume. Her friends mused that she was beginning to age, and medical practitioners were of the opinion that she may have to become accustomed to decreasing performance and energy levels.

The results of this 53 year old female professor G.I. indicate an elevated lead level (three times the high end of normal range) as the most significant finding. In addition, copper is high, thallium is mildly elevated, there is an obvious chromium deficiency and calcium and molybdenum levels are somewhat low.

It was then determined that the water pipes in her residence dated back to the beginning of the 1900's, when they were made of lead! Aside from a prescription similar to the one given to the previous patient, the most important recommendation in this case was to stop using tap water for food preparation or drinking. The water pipes were to be replaced, however this required some time. After a few weeks, fatigue and concentration difficulties disappeared. She returned to her normal self and was able to actively participate in all aspects of her professional and personal life. This treatment represented long-term success.

Case 3 (patient number 1949)
37 year old female (H.R.): Hair mineral analysis

* calcium greater than 2000 ppm and magnesium greater than 200 ppm indicates deficiency status with mobilization of these minerals out of storage (especially from bone)

** ppm = parts per million

Mineral	Reference (ppm)			Test value	Range: Low	Normal	High
Calcium*	350	-	1650	2312		xxxxxxxx	—
Magnesium*	26	-	190	166		xxxxxxxx	
Phosphorous	135	-	275	119	—	xxxxxxxx	
Zinc	190	-	280	249		xxxxxxxx	
Silica	8	-	22	10.6		xxxxxxxx	
Chromium	0.2	-	0.6	< 0.07	——	xxxxxxxx	
Manganese	0.3	-	1.4	0.26	—	xxxxxxxx	
Molybdenum	0.1	-	1.3	< 0.10		xxxxxxxx	
Copper	8	-	48	22.9		xxxxxxxx	
Iron	11	-	24	7.5	—	xxxxxxxx	
Selenium	0.2	-	0.9	< 0.24		xxxxxxxx	
Cobalt	0.1	-	0.3	0.22		xxxxxxxx	
Boron	0	-	3.5	0.33		xxxxxxxx	
Gold	0.2	-	0.5	1.41		xxxxxxxx	——
Silver	0.1	-	0.6	1.31		xxxxxxxx	—
Platinum	0.2	-	0.5	0.40		xxxxxxxx	
Strontium	0.5	-	10	4.72		xxxxxxxx	
Barium	0.4	-	6	15.19		xxxxxxxx	—
Vanadium	0.1	-	0.3	0.33		xxxxxxxx	
Nickel	0.2	-	1.0	0.31		xxxxxxxx	
Germanium	0.2	-	0.4	< 0.31		xxxxxxxx	
Iodine	0	-	22	< 7.1		xxxxxxxx	
Sulfur	31000	-	47000	34053		xxxxxxxx	

Toxic Minerals	Reference range			Test value	Normal	Toxic
Cadmium	0	-	0.6	0.10	xxxxxxx	
Lead	0	-	3.5	< 0.7	xxxxxxx	
Aluminum	0	-	5.0	1.8	xxxxxxx	
Mercury	0	-	2.5	0.90	xxxxxxx	
Arsenic	0	-	3.0	< 1.0	xxxxxxx	

Important laboratory results are in **bold**.
In a comprehensive analysis such as this one, not all minute deviations are significant.

This patient had experienced pain and swelling in practically all skeletal regions for a long time. In the mornings she often felt stiffness, which is typical of inflammatory rheumatism. Several orthopedic clinics were consulted, none of which could offer any help or come up with a conclusive diagnosis. She was a goldsmith by profession and was advised to discontinue her career. She also felt "depleted" psychologically. An orthopedic surgeon referred this patient to one of the authors for analysis.

The most obvious laboratory findings are the significantly elevated gold and silver values, which are two-three times above the higher end values of the normal range. There are also simultaneous chromium and selenium deficiencies as well as milder calcium and molybdenum deficiencies. Increased barium (and often also strontium) levels commonly occur in association with calcium deficiency, and apart from this they have no further significance. This effect seems to occur due to the fact that calcium, barium and strontium all belong to the earth alkali metals (in the same column of the periodic table).

This patient was prescribed all trace elements that had low readings as well as zinc and selenium (which are antagonists to gold and silver and enhance their elimination). Aside from this, she was prescribed 0.5 g of methionine (a sulfur-containing amino acid) twice daily to aid in the elimination of heavy metals. Methionine is conventionally prescribed for the treatment of urinary tract infections.

After two months, this patient discontinued all previous medication for rheumatism. After three months she was symptom-free and decided to discontinue treatment. She thought that her recovery was a miracle, having felt "run down to the ground" before. Feeling as renewed and vigorous as she had been before her illness, she was able to resume bodybuilding and returned to work with newfound enthusiasm and energy.

When her old symptoms mildly returned two years later, they were again successfully eliminated upon renewed treatment. She remained in her career but after knowing the connections she paid particular attention to keep her contact with gold, especially gold dust, as low as possible.

CONCLUSION

This book provides research-based information regarding the theory, practice and limits of using trace minerals in medicine.

Assuming sufficient knowledge and availability of laboratory analysis, the use of trace elements (as well as the vitamins that they work in concert with) can be considered a favorable supplementary treatment approach for many illnesses in terms of effectiveness, side effect risk and cost.

It is relatively rare for a single trace element deficiency to be the sole cause of an illness and for supplementation of this element to be the sole contribution towards alleviating the condition. As a result of current dietary and lifestyle habits, it is much more common for the effects of mild single element deficiencies to gradually intensify over several years (calcium deficiency, for example, develops into osteoporosis after many years). Similarly, poisonous heavy metal exposure from environmental pollution normally accumulates over many years.

An increasing number of illnesses, especially those referred to as "diseases of civilization," are being recognized as having several causative factors. Trace elements can influence these conditions to varying extents.

Trace element therapies are applied most effectively and sensibly in association with conventional medicine. Trace elements are neither universal remedies nor magical solutions. On the other hand, they should not be underrated or considered insignificant.

A situation in which a single measure is sufficient to treat an illness is a fortunate one for everyone involved in the treatment process. However, for many diseases (especially chronic conditions) it is customary in contemporary medicine to employ various treatment approaches simultaneously. For example, surgery on a slipped disc can be followed by physiotherapy in addition to the prescription of drugs (which could include injections and sometimes infusions), without any of these treatments interfering with each other. The type of therapy applied to a particular case is dependent on the available options.

The therapeutic use of trace elements does not represent a competitive threat to other therapies, but can rather be viewed as a supplementary measure with beneficial value varying from case to case.

The initiation of trace element supplementation therapy by practitioners requires start-up time in order to involve laboratory and compounding facilities. The therapies also usually require a higher degree of patient instruction. Financial obligation often remains that of the patient however increasing numbers of insurance companies have extended health care coverage available to medical practitioners including naturopaths, chiropractors, etc.

Patients who have not responded to or have not sufficiently responded to other therapies are the primary users of trace element supplementation. This therapy has repeatedly led to successful results among problem cases. That being said, trace element supplementation should not be considered a universal remedy; it may not be of benefit to every patient. Instead of relying on uncritical and overrated reports, skeptics could be better convinced by qualified statements and case reports of successful therapeutic applications.

Trace elements (and vitamins) are a particularly interesting branch in the growing realm of medical and scientific research. Their therapeutic potential has been underrated. It is hoped that the use of trace elements will become better accepted and integrated into everyday medical practice.

APPENDIX 1

Zinc functions: catalytic, structural, and regulatory roles

It is almost common knowledge that iron is a structural component of hemoglobin, and that iron deficiency can lead to anemia. Most trace elements, however, are required in more than one place within an organism. As an example for this knowledge about the various possible functional mechanisms of trace elements we go into detail concerning zinc.

Even though zinc's importance is often overlooked by some medical practitioners, it has great significance as a trace element and has been intensely researched in the scientific field. The first evidence of zinc's biochemical significance appeared in 1869 for fungi, in 1926 for plants and in 1934 for animals. Over 200 enzymes have been found to contain zinc. The biological functions involving zinc can be divided into categories: catalytic, structural, regulatory, and other functions.

Catalytic functions of zinc

Carbonic anhydrase, discovered in 1940 within red blood cells, catalyzes the reversible hydration reaction of carbon dioxide into carbonic acid. With one atom per molecule, zinc composes only 0.3% of the entire enzyme molecule. Interestingly, the removal of zinc completely inactivates the enzyme even though its structure remains intact. The biological significance and biochemical function of carbonic anhydrase is described at the end of the zinc chapter.

Structural functions of zinc

The requirement for zinc to maintain the structure of certain proteins is referred to as a structural function. Typical examples include the superoxide dismutase and alkaline phosphatase enzymes. Alkaline phosphatase is particularly interesting. It contains four zinc atoms per molecule – two have structural functions and the other two have catalytic functions. This is an example of different action mechanisms working within the same protein molecule. In experiments, serum alkaline phosphatase activity in rats was reduced by 25% after two days of zinc deficiency. After four days, its activity dropped to 50%. As a result of zinc supplementation, alkaline phosphatase activity was restored to the level observed in a control group within three days. The activation of alkaline phosphatase is specific to zinc and is therefore used as an indicator of zinc deficiency in blood tests.

Regulatory functions of zinc

Zinc carries out a regulatory function in fructose-1,6-biphosphatase by affecting activation or inhibition without being required for the enzyme's activity itself. Experimentally, it is difficult to examine these types of regulatory functions.

Other biological functions of zinc

Even though there has been much focus on zinc as a component of enzymes, it also plays other structural and functional roles:

- Zinc is important for the structure and function of biological and plasma membranes. This explains why zinc deficiency in rats leads to decreased resistance to hemolysis of erythrocyte membranes in hypotonic solutions.
- Zinc plays a role in hormones. It is used in the production, storage and release of insulin and sex hormones, as well as in the activation of hormone receptors.
- Zinc is involved in nucleic acid and protein metabolism, cell differentiation, and cell division. Bound zinc stabilizes the structure of RNA, DNA and ribosomes. Many "lock and key" enzymes involved in the synthesis and degradation of nucleic acids, such as thymidine kinase, DNA and RNA polymerase, reverse transcriptase and ribonuclease, are zinc-dependent.
- Zinc is important for proper immune system function.
- Several proteins that are zinc-dependent or that contain zinc do not have any enzymatic properties but take part in many metabolic processes (e.g. metallothionein).

Zinc deficiency symptons

All this information describes the diverse places of action of zinc in biological events. The extent of zinc deficiency symptoms cannot simply be explained by considering the symptoms that would arise from the malfunction of all of the 200 known zinc enzymes. In cases of zinc deficiency, other significant factors play a role, such as, how tightly zinc is bound to an enzyme or how long the enzyme molecule remains active before it is degraded.

When bound loosely, zinc is lost very easily. Some enzymes are very sensitive and deactivate quickly while others are hardly affected even if a deficiency is quite severe. An enzyme with a long lifespan, for example, is affected only by chronic deficiency states.

The chemical and physical properties of zinc, including its position on the periodic table of elements, will be discussed briefly. Similar principles, not described here, can be applied to determine the chemical and physical properties of other trace elements.

Like many essential trace elements (such as iron, cobalt, nickel, copper, chromium and manganese), zinc belongs to the transitional elements in period 4 (the fourth row of the periodic table). Its specific chemical properties are a result of its electron configuration. As a IIB element it has a full 3d electron shell and two 4s electrons, therefore it should actually no longer be a transitional element. Unlike copper or iron, zinc cannot donate an electron from its d-shell and therefore does not take part in metabolic redox reactions. However, zinc is similar to many other trace elements in that it can readily form complexes with various organic compounds found in the body. This is due to its charge and relatively small ionic radius. For this reason, zinc is primarily found in tissues and body fluids in the form of complexes and only exists as a free ion under limited circumstances. Due to electron configuration, zinc compounds are colorless – as opposed to red iron compounds and blue copper-binding proteins. This is probably why zinc's biological significance was discovered so late.

While zinc is an essential element, some of the more toxic elements in the periodic table are found in its vicinity: cadmium is directly underneath, while lead is two rows beneath zinc.

Clinical assessment of trace mineral status is not solely determined by deficiency or excess symptoms. From the example of zinc above, one can apply similar principles and determine the properties that other trace elements have on their own or in relation to other elements. This inter-relationship should be regarded for the therapeutical application.

APPENDIX 2

Radioactive isotopes

Radioactive isotopes derived secondary to nuclear accidents (including the Chernobyl disaster, and atomic/nuclear bomb testing) are described in the following tables.

Most significant radioactive isotopes		
Isotope	**Half life**	**Target organs / specific effects**
Yttrium-90*	3 days	liver, pancreas, reproductive gland
Iodine-131	8 days	thyroid gland, thyroid cancer
Krypton-85	10 years	fatty tissues, cancer risk
Tritium H3	12 years	cancer risk, damage to the fetus
Strontium-90	28 years	bones, bone marrow damage, leukemia
Cesium-137	33 years	muscels, cancer risk
Carbon-14	5700 years	chromosomal damage, cancer risk
Plutonium-239	24,000 years	lungs, lung cancer
Iodine-129	11 million years	same as Iodine-131

*by-product of strontium-90 decay.

- **Carbon-14** is dispersed through the air and accumulates in the food chain. Since it can be incorporated into all organic compounds, it can cause significant damage.
- **Cesium-137** can also be accumulated by plants. Another isotope, cesium-134, has a half-life of 2 years.
- **Iodine-129/131** disrupts growth in children. Since it has an affinity for reproductive glands, it can lead to future hereditary changes.
- **Krypton-85** is a noble gas and extremely difficult to filter out. Since it is heavier than air, it stays low to the ground and is absorbed by plants. It is also soluble in body fluids.
- **Plutonium-239** is probably the most poisonous chemical element on earth. It is believed that 500 g of plutonium evenly distributed throughout the earth's atmosphere could elicit 9 billion cases of lung cancer. Plutonium is the basic element used in the construction of atomic bombs.
- **Strontium-90** is a component of radioactive fallout. It is absorbed by plants, eaten by cows, and then ingested by humans via cow's milk.

Strontium-89 is also radioactive.

- **Tritium H3** is radioactive hydrogen. When reacting with oxygen to form water, it can enter all body cells. Cells are composed primarily of water. Tritium is also incorporated into chromosomes. As a gas, it can penetrate steel, concrete and other building materials and therefore emanate from containers and tanks.
- Other radioactive isotopes and their half-lives include tellurium-132 (3 days) and 131, ruthenium-103 (39 days) and 106 (1 year), barium-140, molybdenum-99 and technetium-99.

In total, about 200 isotopes of 35-40 different elements are found in radioactive fall-out. They have the same biological properties and target organs as their natural counterparts, yet cause extensive damage due to their radioactivity. Further, differences exist between the effects of alpha, beta and gamma radiation.

The symptoms of radiation sickness become apparent when cell division is disrupted (and eventually stops). The first signs originate from the gastric area and can be identified by bleeding and diarrhea. After some time, the bone marrow is affected, resulting in anemia and immune weakness.

While this acute phase reaches its peak within a few weeks or months, the risk of various cancers rises after several years. In many cases it takes several decades.

Nuclear weapon testing "in the atmosphere" was not uncommon several decades ago. The end result is environmental worldwide radioactive exposure.

REFERENCES

The following list includes some particularly interesting journals, as well as various books. English publications, followed by German ones, are presented in alphabetical order according to author names.

Journals:

Biological Trace Element Research. Humana Press Inc. ISSN 0163-4984 (monthly) Example: (Volume 24-Number 2), Feb. 1990.

The Journal of Applied Nutrition. International College of Applied Nutrition. ISSN 0021-8960.

Journal of Orthomolecular Medicine (JOM). ISSN 0317-0209. (quarterly)

Journal of Trace Elements in Medicine and Biology. Stuttgart (and GMS): Gustav-Fischer-Verlag. ISSN 0946-672X. Example: March 1995.

Magnesium Bulletin. Heidelberg: Verlag fuer Medizin. ISSN 0172-908X. (quarterly)

Vita Min Spur/Vitamin-Minerals-Trace elements. Stuttgart: Hippocrates Verlag, ISSN 0930-4827. (quarterly) (Since 1995, this journal has been succeeded by the *Journal of Trace Elements in Medicine and Biology*, above.)

Books:

Bosco, D. *The People's Guide to Vitamins and Minerals, from A to Zinc.* Chicago: Contemporary books, 1989. ISBN 0-8092-4582-5

Chatt, A. and Katz, S. *Hair Analysis.* New York: VCH Publishers Inc., 10010 (1988), ISBN 3-527-26787-5: VCH-Verlagsgesellschaft. ISBN 3-527-26787-5

Foster, H. *What Really Causes AIDS.* Victoria, British Columbia: Trafford, 2002. ISBN 155369132-6.

Hendler, S., M.D., Ph.D. *The Doctor's Vitamin and Mineral Encyclopedia.* New York: Simon and Schuster, 1990. ISBN 0-671-66784-X

Hoffer, A., M.D., Ph.D. *Orthomolecular Medicine for Physicians.* Connecticut: Keats Publishing Inc., 1989. ISBN 0-87933-390-4.

Hoffer, A, M.D., Ph.D. *Dr. Hoffer's ABC of Natural Nutrition for Children.* Quarry Press Inc., 1999. ISBN 1-55082-185-7.

Hoffer, A., M.D., Ph.D. and Walker, M., D.P.M. *Orthomolecular Nutrition.* Connecticut: Keats Publishing Inc., 1987.

Hoffer, A., M.D., Ph.D. and Walker, M., D.P.M. *Putting it all Together, the New Orthomolecular Nutrition.* Connecticut: Keats Publishing Inc., 1996. ISBN 0-87983-633-4.

Pfeiffer, CC. *Mental and Elemental Nutrients: a Physician's Guide to Nutrition and Health Care.* Connecticut: Keats Publishing Inc., 1975. ISBN 0-87983-114-6.

Pfeiffer, CC. *Zinc and Other Micro-Nutrients.* Connecticut: Keats Publishing Inc., 1978. ISBN 0-87983-169-3.

Pfeiffer, CC. *Zinc and Other Micro-Nutrients.* Connecticut: Keats Publishing Inc., 1987, pp. 66-73.

Schrauzer, G. *Selenium.* Clifton, New Jersey: Humana Press, 1988. ISBN 0-89603-154-3.

Werbach, M., M.D. *Nutritional Influences on Illness.* Tarzana, California: Third Line Press Inc., 1991. ISBN 0-9618550-0-2.
2nd Ed: 1993. ISBN 0-9618550-3-7.

Werbach, M., M.D. *Nutritional Influences on Mental Illness.* Tarzana, California: Third Line Press Inc., 1991. ISBN 0-9618550-1-0.

Braetter, P. and Gramm, H.-J. *Mineralstoffe und Spurenelemente in der Ernaehrung des Menschen.* Berlin: Blackwell, Wissenschafts-Verlag, 1991. ISBN 3-89412-115-7.

Burgerstein, L. *Heilwirkung von Naehrstoffen.* 7th ed. Heidelberg: Haug Verlag, 1994. ISBN 3-7760-0989-6. The 8th edition (below) was completely reworked and expanded.

Burgerstein, L. *Handbuch Naehrstoffe.* 8th ed. Heidelberg: Haug Verlag, 1997. ISBN 3-7760-1666-3. The 8th edition was completely reworked and expanded.

Daunderer, M. *Handbuch der Umweltgifte 1, 2, 3, 4* (binder package). Landsberg: Ecomed Verlagsgesellschaft, updated regularly. ISBN 3-609-71136-1.

Daunderer, M. Amalgamated special edition of *Klinische Toxikologie.* Landsberg: Ecomed Verlagsgesellschaft. ISBN 3-609-70016-5.

Holtmeister, K.-J. *Zink.* Stuttgart: Wissenschaftliche Verlagsgesellschaft, 1991. ISBN 3-8047-0898-6

"Gesellschaft fuer Mineralstoffe und Spurenelemente." (GMS: Association for Minerals and Trace Minerals, where one of the authors has been a longstanding member. GMS has also published other books.)

Upon further interest in this subject, specialized literature can be obtained through the literature listed above, and through **specialized libraries** such as:

- Stiftung zur Internationalen Foerderung der Orthomolekularen Medizin, Postfach CH-8640 Rapperswil.
- Zentralbibliothek der Medizin Koeln, Joseph-Stelzmann-Str. 9, Tel.: 0221/478-5608.

On the **internet:**

- DIMDI (Deutsches Institut fuer Medizinische Dokumentation und Information). Available at: http://www.dimdi.de/qui.html.
- The Linus Pauling Institute Available at: http://lpi.oregonstate.edu.

OTHER REFERENCES

Anderson RA. Chromium metabolism and its role in disease processes in men. *Clinical Physiology and Biochemistry.* 4:31-41, 1986.

Arsenian, M. A. Magnesium and cardiovascular disease. *Prog. in Cardiovascular Disease* 35: 271-310, 1993.

Bates C.J., Powers H.J. and Thurnham D.I. Vitamins, iron and physical work. *The Lancet.* 2: 313-314, 1989.

Becker DV et al., The use of iodone as a thyroidal blocking agent in the event of a reactor accident. *Journal of the American Medical Association.* 252:659-661, 1984.

Benton, D. and Buts, J.P. Vitamin/mineral supplementation and intelligence. *The Lancet,* 1: 1158-1160, 1990.

Benton, D. and Cook, R. The impact of selenium supplementation on mood. *Biological Psychiatry.* 29: 1092-1098, 1991.

Benton, D., Haller, J., and Fordy, J. Vitamin supplementation for one year improves mood. *Neuropsychobiology.* 32: 98-105, 1995.

Benton, D. and Roberts, G. Effect of vitamin and mineral supplementation on intelligence of a sample of school children. *The Lancet.* 1: 140-143, 1988.

Carlisle EM. The Nutritional essentiality of silicon. *Nutrition Reviews.* 40: 193-198, 1982.

Cetinkaya, N. and Cetinkaya, D. Serum copper, zinc levels and copper zinc ratio in healthy women and women with gynecological tumors. *Biological Trace Element Research.* 18: 29-38, 1988.

Dale G et al. Fitness, unfitness and phosphate. *British Medicine Journal*. 294: 939, 1987.

Dallman P.R. Iron deficiency and the immune response. *American Journal of Clinical Nutrition*. 46: 329-334, 1987.

Dubey A and Solomon R. Magnesium, myocardial ischaemia and arrhythmias: The role of magnesium in myocardial infarction. *Drugs*. 37: 1-7, 1989.

Dworkin BM et al. Selenium deficiency in the acquired immunodeficiency syndrome. *Journal of Parenteral Nutrition*. 10: 405-407, 1986.

Freeland-Graves JH. Manganese: An essential nutrient for humans. *Nutrition Today*. Nov-Dec: 13-19, 1988.

Friedman B.J. et al. Manganese: balance and clinical observations in young men fed a manganese-deficient diet. *Journal of Nutrition*. 117: 133-143, 1987.

Goode, H.F., Kelleher, J., Walker, B.E., Hall, R.I., and Guillou, P.I. Cellular and muscle zinc in surgical patients with and without gastrointestinal cancer. *Clinical Science*. 79: 247-252, 1990.

Gottschalk, L.A. , Rebello, T., Buchsbaum, M.S., Tucker, H.G., and Hodges, E.L. Abnormalities in hair trace elements as indicators of aberrant behavior. *Comprehensive Psychiatry*. 23: 229-237, 1991.

Jeejeebhoy KN et al. Chromium deficiency, glucose intolerance and neuropathy reversed by chromium supplementation in a patient receiving long-term total parenteral nutrition. *American Journal of Clinical Nutrition*. 3: 531-538, 1977.

Jenner, P. Oxidative damage in neurodegenerative disease. *The Lancet*. 344: 796-798, 1994.

Khaw K-T and Barrett-Connor E. Dietary potassium and stroke-associated mortality: a 12-year prospective population study. *New England Journal of Medicine*. 316: 325-240, 1987.

Kok FJ et al. Decreased selenium levels in acute myocardial infarction. *Journal of the American Medical Association*. 261: 1161-1164, 1989.

Look, M.P. Sodium selenite and N-acetylcysteine in antiretroviral-naive HIV-1 infected patients: a randomized controlled pilot study. *European Journal of Clinical Investigation*. 28(5): 389-397, 1998.

Naylor G.J. Vanadium and manic-depressive psychosis. *Nutrition and Health*. 3: 79, 1984.

Nelson, P., Naismith, D.J., Burley, J., Gatenby, S., and Geddes, N. Nutrient intake vitamin/mineral supplementation and intelligence in British school children. *British Journal of Nutrition*. 64: 13-22, 1989.

Newsome DA et al. Oral zinc in macular degeneration. *Archives of Ophthalmology.* 106: 192-198, 1988.

Nielsen F.H. Boron: an overlooked element of potential nutritional importance. *Nutrition Today.* Jan-Feb: 4-7, 1988.

Nielsen F.H. et al. Effect of dietary boron on mineral, estrogen, and testosterone metabolism in postmenopausal women. *Federation of American Societies for Experimental Biology (FASEB) Journal.* 1: 394-397, 1987.

Press R.I., Geller J. and Evans G.W. The effect of chromium picolinate on serum cholesterol and apolipoprotein fractions in human subjects. *Western Journal of Medicine.* 152: 41-45, 1990.

Rajagopalan K.V. Molybdenum: An essential trace element in human nutrition. *Annual Review of Nutrition.* 8: 401-427, 1988.

Rasmussen H.S. et al. Intravenous magnesium in acute myocardial infarction. *The Lancet.* 1: 234-235, 1986.

Salonen J.T. et al. Association between cardiovascular death and myocardial infarction and serum selenium in a matched-pair longitudinal study. *The Lancet.* 2: 175, 1982.

Sjogren A., Edvinsson L. and Fallgren B., Magnesium deficiency in coronary artery disease and cardiac arrhythmias. *Journal of Internal Medicine.* 226: 213-222, 1989.

U.S. Congress, Office of Technology Assessment. Neurotoxicity: Identifying and Controlling Poisons of the Nervous System. U. S. Government Printing Office, publication #OTA-BA-436, 1990.

Walsh, William J., PhD. Zinc deficiency, metal metabolism, and behavior disorders: a Report of the Health Research Institute. Naperville, IL, March, 1996.

Walsh, W.J., Usman, A., Tarpey, J, and Kelly, T. Metallothionein and Autism. Naperville, Illinois: Pfeiffer Treatment Center, 2001(October).

Walter T., Kovalskys J. and Stekel A.L. Effect of mild iron deficiency on infant mental development scores. *Journal of Pediatrics.* 102: 510-522, 1983.

Whang, Robert. Electrolyte and water metabolism in sports activities. *Comprehensive Therapy.* 24: 5-8, 1998 (January).

Williams D.M. Copper deficiency in humans. *Seminars in Hematology.* 20: 118-128, 1983.

Yu. S.; Mai, B., Xiao, P., Yu, W., Wang, Y., Huang, C., Chen, W., and Xuan, X. Intervention trial with selenium for the prevention of lung cancer among tin miners in Yunnan, China: a pilot study. *Biological Trace Element Research.* 24: 105-108, 1990.

The Periodic Table of the Elements

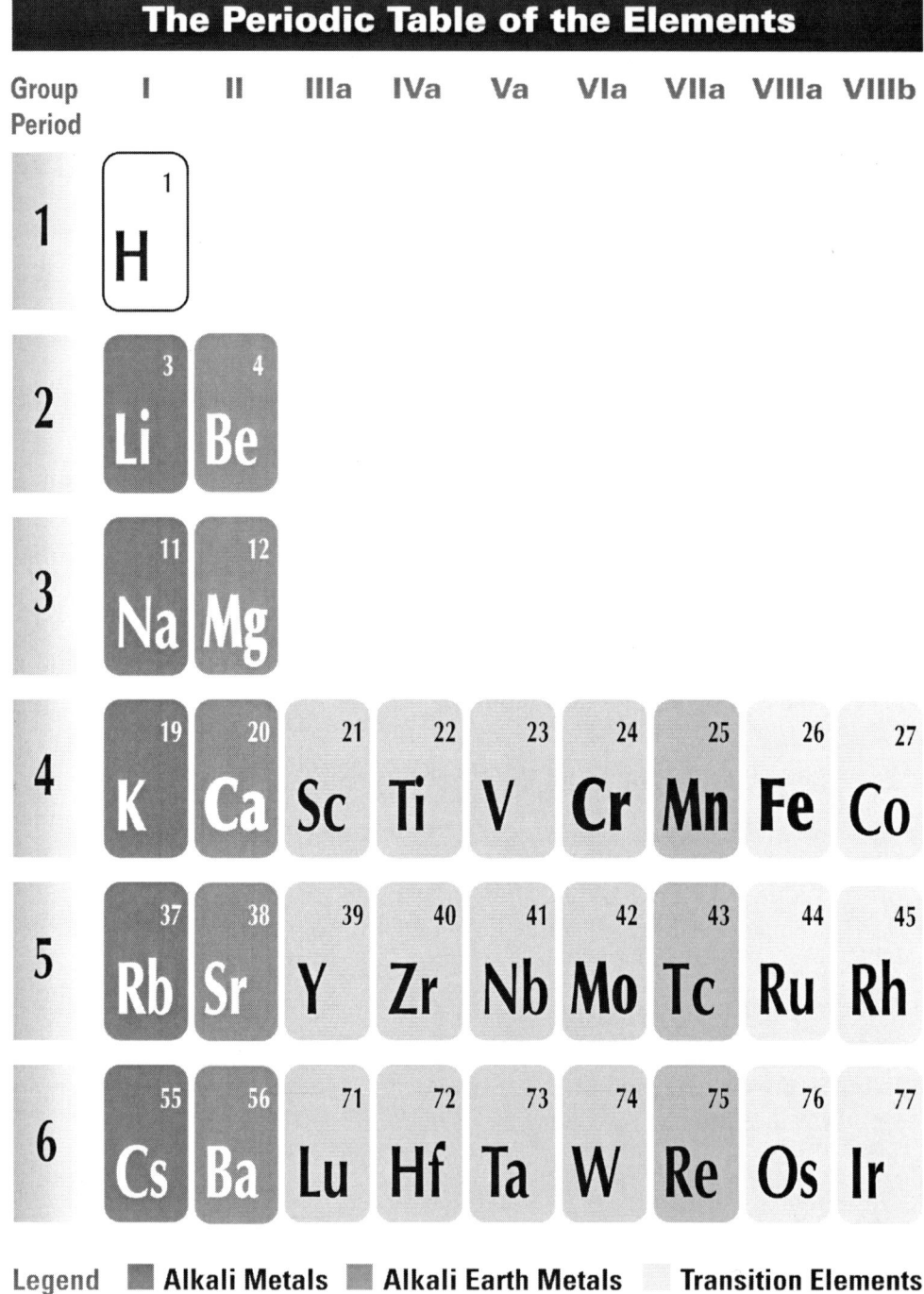

Group Period	I	II	IIIa	IVa	Va	VIa	VIIa	VIIIa	VIIIb
1	1 H								
2	3 Li	4 Be							
3	11 Na	12 Mg							
4	19 K	20 Ca	21 Sc	22 Ti	23 V	24 Cr	25 Mn	26 Fe	27 Co
5	37 Rb	38 Sr	39 Y	40 Zr	41 Nb	42 Mo	43 Tc	44 Ru	45 Rh
6	55 Cs	56 Ba	71 Lu	72 Hf	73 Ta	74 W	75 Re	76 Os	77 Ir

Legend ■ Alkali Metals ■ Alkali Earth Metals ▫ Transition Elements

The Periodic Table of Elements

The number in the upper right of each box designates that element's atomic number. The group number of an element tells us the number of electrons

The Periodic Table of the Elements

VIIIc	IB	IIB	III	IV	V	VI	VII	VIII
								2 He
			5 B	6 C	7 N	8 O	9 F	10 Ne
			13 Al	14 Si	15 P	16 S	17 Cl	18 Ar
28 Ni	29 Cu	30 Zn	31 Ga	32 Ge	33 As	34 Se	35 Br	36 Kr
46 Pd	47 Ag	48 Cd	49 In	50 Sn	51 Sb	52 Te	53 I	54 Xe
78 Pt	79 Au	80 Hg	81 Tl	82 Pb	83 Bi	84 Po	85 At	86 Rn

Group III-VI   Halogens   Noble Gases

in the outer shell. Transition elements have bio-chemically significant catalytic properties.

INDEX

This index is designed for quick desktop reference. There are a comprehensive array of search terms. To narrow your search, keywords are referenced by page number, followed by a parentheses () containing the element chapter and chapter page number. Page 125 (Zn12), for example, refers to page 125 of the book and page 12 of the Zinc (Zn) chapter. **f** includes the following page, **ff** includes 2 or more of the following pages, and **>>** points to another index-word.

A

Acid/base regulation, 28 (Cd3), 60 (K1f), 124 (Zn11f), 150

Acid rain, xiii, 93 (S2), 98 (Se3), 109 (Tl2)

Acrodermatitis enteropathica, 116 (Zn3+7+10)

ADD/ADHD, 39 (Cu4), 43 (F2), 55 (Hg6), 84 (P1f), 88 (Pb3), 119 (Zn6) >> concentration, memory, brain

Adolescents, 43 (F2), 73 (Mn1), 98 (Se3), 115 (Zn2,4+6)

Aging, 40 (Cu5), 73 (Mn1), 89 (Pb4), 96 (Se1), 121 (Zn8+10), 128, 135, 145 >> free radicals

Aggression, 38 (Cu3), 87 (Pb2)

Airborne particles/gases, 5 (Al2), 8 (As3), 15 (Ba2), 17 (Be2), 21 (Br2), 27 (Cd2+4), 33 (Co2), 35 (Cr2), 40 (Cu5), 44 (F3), 51 (Hg2ff+6), 90 (Pt1f), 93 (S2), 102 (Si1f), 105 (Sn2), 147, 153

Alcohol, 12 (B1f), 25 (Ca4), 31 (Cl2), 71 (Mg6f), 96 (Se1+6), 117 (Zn4ff)

Alkaline phosphatase, 28 (Cd3), 123 (Zn10ff), 150

Allergies, 12 (B1f), 20 (Br1f), 22 (Ca1ff), 35 (Cr2), 50 (Hg1+5), 58 (I3f), 73 (Mn1f), 82 (Ni1f), 85 (P2), 90 (Pt1f)

ALS (amyotrophic lateral sclerosis), 75 (Mn3), 101 (Se6)

Alzheimer's disease, 4 (Al1f), 77 (Mo2), 101 (Se6), 122 (Zn9)

Aluminum, 4 (Al1f), 85 (P2), 129, 136

Amalgams, >> dental

Amines, biogenic, 37 (Cu2), 121 (Zn8) >> catecholamines

Amino acids

    cysteine, 4 (Al1), 6 (As1), 77 (Mo2), 93 (S2), 121 (Zn8)

    general considerations, 35 (Cr2), 37 (Cu2), 67 (Mg2), 91 (Pt2), 121 (Zn8), 132

    glutamate (glutamic acid), 65 (Li4), 121 (Zn8f)

    homocysteine, 77 (Mo2), 93 (S2)

    lysine (and lysine monooxygenase), 37 (Cu2)

    metabolism of, 35 (Cr2), 67 (Mg2), 91 (Pt2), 121 (Zn8)

    methionine, 93 (S2), 147

    receptors (NMDA), 121 (Zn8)

    sulfur-containing, 4 (Al1f), 6 (As1), 12 (B1), 26 (Cd1), 52 (Hg3), 77 (Mo2), 86 (Pb1), 92 (S1f), 121 (Zn8), 147

Anemia, 11 (Au2), 32 (Co1f), 46 (Fe2), 78 (Mo3), 86 (Pb1ff), 100 (Se5), 115 (Zn2), 133f, 150, 154

Anorexia, 25 (Ca4), 59 (I4), 60 (K1f), 66 (Mg1), 112 (V1), 117 (Zn4), 121 (Zn8f)

Antagonistic elements, >> copper-zinc-manganese-molybdenum-antagonism, calcium-antagonists

Antimony, 94 (Sb1f)

Antioxidants, >> free radicals

Arachidonic acid, 64 (Li3), 100 (Se5) >> prostaglandin metabolism

Arsenic, xiif, 6 (As1-4), 40 (Cu5), 53 (Hg4), 95 (Sb2), 97 (Se2), 130f

Arteries, >> blood

Arteriosclerosis, 75 (Mn3), 77 (Mo2), 100 (Se5f), 124 (Zn11)

Diabetes, 35 (Cr2), 47 (Fe3), 72 (Mg7), 73-74 (Mn1-2), 96 (Se1), 112 (V1), 117 (Zn4-11)

Diarrhea, 6 (As1+3), 13 (B2), 14 (Ba1f), 28 (Cd3f), 31 (Cl2), 40 (Cu5), 44 (F3), 52 (Hg3), 60 (K1), 62 (Li1f), 66 (Mg1), 80 (Na1f), 95 (Sb2), 105 (Sn2), 109 (Tl2), 118 (Zn5), 138, 154

E

Ear, 73 (Mn1), 123 (Zn10)

Eczema (and atopic dermatitis), 8 (As3), 16 (Be1), 19 (Bi2), 35 (Cr2), 38 (Cu3), 59 (I4), 64 (Li3), 90 (Pt1f), 121 (Zn8)

Elastin, 37 (Cu2) >> collagen

Elderly, xiv, 13 (B2), 40 (Cu5), 69 (Mg4), 73 (Mn1), 101 (Se6), 117 (Zn4+8f), 121 (Zn8), 134f >> aging

Emissions, compare airborne particles/ gases

    automobile, 26 (Cd1), 86 (Pb1f), 90 (Pt1f)

    industrial, 7 (As2), 27 (Cd2), 29 (Cd4), 32 (Co1)

Energy, 49 (Ge2), 57 (I2), 84 (P1f), 124 (Zn11), 145, 147 >> fatigue

Environmental protection, 24 (Ca3), 27 (Cd2ff), 51 (Hg2+6), 89 (Pb4), 110 (Tl3) >> pollution, radiation

Enzymes

    activators, 61 (K2), 66 (Mg1f), 73 (Mn1), 91 (Pt2)

    alcohol dehydrogenase, 122 (Zn9ff)

    aldehyde oxidase, 76 (Mo1f)

    alkaline phosphatase, 28 (Cd3), 123 (Zn10), 125 (Zn12), 150

    amino-oxidase, 37 (Cu2)

    carbonic anhydrase (CA), 115 (Zn2+11f), 150

    citric acid cycle, 73 (Mn1)

    cytochrome oxidase, 37 (Cu2)

    dopamine-beta-hydroxylase, 37 (Cu2)

    ferro-oxidase II, 37 (Cu2)

    glutamate decarboxylase (and dehydrogenase), 121 (Zn8f)

    glutathionperoxidase, 100 (Se5)

    glutamine synthetase, 122 (Zn9)

    lysine monooxygenase, 37 (Cu2)

    malate dehydrogenase, 73 (Mn1)

    mineral enzymes, 33 (Co2), 36 (Cu1), 61 (K2), 66 (Mg1f), 73 (Mn1f), 76 (Mo1), 114 (Zn1), 150f

    monoamine oxidase (MAO), 36 (Cu1)

    nitrate reductase, 78 (Mo3)

    ornithine carbamoyl transferase, 122 (Zn9)

    pyruvate carboxylase, 73 (Mn1)

    prolidase, 75 (Mn3)

    prolylhydroxylase, 103 (Si2)

    sulfite oxidase, 76 (Mo1f)

    superoxide dismutase (SOD), >> superoxide dismutase

    thyroid hormone type-I-5´ deiodase, 59 (I4), 100 (Se5)

    tyrosinase, 37 (Cu2)

    urease, 82 (Ni1f), 122 (Zn9), 125 (Zn12)

    vitamin B12 related, 33 (Co2)

    xanthine dehydrogenase, 77 (Mo2)

    xanthine oxidase, 76 (Mo1f)

    zinc-containing, 115 (Zn2), 121-122 (Zn8-9), 125 (Zn12), 150-151

Epilepsy, 19 (Bi2), 20 (Br1f), 72 (Mg7)

Estrogen, 13 (B2), 24 (Ca3), 39 (Cu4), 71 (Mg6), 73 (Mn1), 78 (Mo3), 85 (P2), 124 (Zn11)

Excretion

    intestines (stool), via, 5 (Al2), 8 (As3), 38 (Cu3), 45 (Fe1), 52 (Hg3ff), 61 (K2), 63 (Li2), 109 (Tl2)

    kidneys (urine), via, 5 (Al2), 8 (As3), 11 (Au2), 24 (Ca3), 27 (Cd2ff), 31 (Cl2), 35 (Cr2), 44 (F3), 49 (Ge2), 61 (K2), 63 (Li2), 67 (Mg2ff), 71 (Mg6f), 85 (P2), 88 (Pb6), 93 (S2), 103 (Si2), 109 (Tl2), 118 (Zn5)

    perspiration, via, 35 (Cr2), 45 (Fe1), 63 (Li2), 67 (Mg2), 118 (Zn5)

Exercise and physical ability, 31 (Cl2), 60 (K1f), 64 (Li3), 67 (Mg2), 70 (Mg5f), 85 (Pb2), 87 (Pb2), 114 (Zn1ff), 134, 139 >> muscles

F

Fats/lipids, xiv, 34 (Cr1f), 72 (Mg7), 83 (Ni2), 90 (Pt1), 112 (V1)

76 (Mo1f), 90 (Pt1f), 96 (Se1f+5f), 114 (Zn1f+1), 135, 141 >> peroxidation

G

GABA, 121 (Zn8)
Gall bladder, 66 (Mg1), 70 (Mg5), 118 (Zn5)
Garbage incineration, 27 (Cd2+4), 51 (Hg2)
Garlic odor, 7 (As2), 97 (Se2)
Genetic disturbances/disorders, 17 (Be2), 38 (Cu3), 59 (I4), 75 (Mn3), 101 (Se6), 116 (Zn3+6+11)
Germanium, 48 (Ge1f)
Glucose tolerance factor (GTF), 34 (Cr1f)
Glutathione, vi, 59 (I4), 96 (Se1+5), 135
Glutathionperoxidase, 100 (Se5)
Gold, 3 (Ag2), 10 (Au1f), 53 (Hg4+6), 147
Gout, 12 (B1), 77 (Mo2)
Growth and development, xiv, 22 (Ca1f), 36 (Cu1+3+5), 45 (Fe1ff), 56 (I1ff), 72 (Mg7), 84 (P1), 88 (Pb3), 105 (Sn2), 114 (Zn1f+6f), 134, 153

H

Hair, >> collagen
  alopecia areata, 121 (Zn8)
  brittle, 45 (Fe1)
  coarse hair, 37 (Cu2)
  color, 36 (Cu1f)
  dye/bleach/perm, 82 (Ni1f),
  elasticity, 36 (Cu1), 103 (Si2), 130
  element storage/deposition, 7 (As2f), 40 (Cu5), 109 (Tl2), 117 (Zn4), 128f, 132
  forensic evaluation, 128, 130
  growth/structure, 25 (Ca4), 36 (Cu1f), 92 (S1f), 97 (Se2), 103 (Si2), 119 (Zn6)
  keratin, 93 (S2), 121 (Zn8)
  kinky hair, 40 (Cu5)
  loss, 6 (As1+3), 37 (Cu2), 76 (Mo1), 97 (Se2), 105 (Sn2), 109 (Tl2), 114 (Zn1+3+7f)
  mental, 38 (Cu3), 55 (Hg6), 56 (I1f), 75 (Mn3), 76 (Mo1), 86 (Pb1f), 114 (Zn1f+6+9) >> brain
Hair mineral analysis, 5 (Al2), 7 (As2), 40 (Cu5), 53 (Hg4), 59 (I4), 68 (Mg3), 75 (Mn3), 125 (Zn12), 128ff

pubic versus head hair, 109 (Tl2), 119 (Zn6), 133
  sweat confound, 35 (Cr2), 83 (Ni2), 118 (Zn5), 132f
Headaches, 3 (Ag2), 29 (Cd4), 39 (Cu4), 45 (Fe1), 52 (Hg3+5), 68 (Mg3f), 83 (Ni2), 88 (Pb3), 93 (S2), 95 (Sb2), 97 (Se2), 105 (Sn2) >> migraine
Heart, >> muscle
  angina, 26 (Cd1), 47 (Fe3), 69 (Mg4), 77 (Mo2), 80 (Na1f), 96 (Se1+3f), 112 (V1f), 117 (Zn4f+12)
  disease/damage, 16 (Be1f), 26 (Cd1), 62 (Li1f)
  medications, 24 (Ca3), 60 (K1), 69 (Mg4), 99 (Se4)
  mineral storage/deposition, 24 (Ca3), 37 (Cu2), 69 (Mg4), 100 (Se5), 117 (Zn4)
  rhythm disturbance, 14 (Ba1f), 47 (Fe3), 60 (K1f), 66 (Mg1), 69 (Mg4), 125 (Zn12)
Heavy metals
  absorption/deposition, 24 (Ca3), 98 (Se3), 111 (Zn1ff), 132, 135, 148
  removal/excretion, 2 (Ag1), 4 (Al1f), 6 (As1), 24 (Ca3), 26 (Cd1ff), 38 (Cu3f), 47 (Fe3), 48 (Ge1f), 50 (Hg1+3ff), 77 (Mo2f), 86 (Pb1), 90 (Pt1), 92 (S1f), 96 (Se1+4ff), 111 (Zn1+11), 129, 135f, 140, 147, 152
  sources and exposures, 2 (Ag1f), 4 (Al1f), 6 (As1ff), 16 (Be1f), 18 (Bi1f), 26 (Cd1), 32 (Co1f), 36 (Cu1+5), 46 (Fe2), 50 (Hg1-3+6), 74 (Mn2f), 82 (Ni1f), 86 (Pb1ff), 90 (Pt1f), 98 (Se3), 104 (Sn1f), 111, 132, 148
Heidelberg-Emmertsgrund, 108-109 (Tl1-2)
Hemochromatosis, 47 (Fe3), 136
Histamine, 31 (Cl2), 73 (Mn1), 121 (Zn8) >> amines
Horton's neuralgia, 62 (Li1+3)
Hydrogen, 124-125 (Zn11-12), 153
Hyperimidodipeptidurea (prolidase deficiency), 75 (Mn3)

I

Immune system, 12 (B1f), 23 (Ca2), 28 (Cd3), 40 (Cu5), 46 (Fe2), 48 (Ge1f), 52 (Hg3f), 64 (Li3), 73 (Mn1f), 83 (Ni2),

91 (Pt2), 96 (Se1ff), 102 (Si1f), 114 (Zn1ff+11))

Industrial waste, 3 (Ag2), 27 (Cd2ff), 52 (Hg3), 82 (Ni1f), 108 (Tl1ff)

Infants/newborns, 3 (Ag2), 22 (Ca1f), 27 (Cd2), 43 (F2f), 47 (Fe3), 56 (I1f), 60 (K1), 71 (Mg6f), 77 (Mo2), 85 (P2), 88 (Pb3), 101 (Se6), 114 (Zn1+4+6), 137 >> pregnancy

Infection
  acute, 40 (Cu5), 118 (Zn5)
  chronic, 34 (Cr1), 49 (Ge2), 96 (Se1+5), 117 (Zn4f+10)
  susceptibility, v, 40 (Cu5), 45 (Fe1f), 50 (Hg1+5), 64 (Li3), 75 (Mn3), 88 (Pb3), 91 (Pt2), 101 (Se6), 117 (Zn4), 135

Insulin, 34 (Cr1f), 82 (Ni1f), 85 (P2), 113 (V2), 117 (Zn4+11), 151

Intrinsic factor, >> stomach

Iodine, xiif, xvf, 21 (Br2), 24 (Ca3), 33 (Co2), 43 (F2), 56 (I1ff), 64 (Li3), 81 (Na2), 100 (Se5f), 107 (Sr2), 129, 153

Iodine antagonists, 43 (F2), 56 (I1)

IQ, 43 (F2), 78 (Mo3), 88 (Pb3) >> ADD, memory

Iron, xii-xiv, xvi, 25 (Ca4), 28 (Cd3), 36 (Cu1f+5), 45 (Fe1ff), 54 (Hg5), 59 (I4), 67 (Mg2), 72 (Mg7), 73 (Mn1), 78 (Mo3), 85 (P2), 113 (V2), 115 (Zn2), 128ff, 141, 150f

Iron overload, >> hemochromatosis

Itai-Itai disease, 28 (Cd3)

J

Joints/arthritis, 2 (Ag1f), 10 (Au1f), 12 (B1), 17 (Be2), 26 (Cd1ff), 40 (Cu5), 47 (Fe3), 48 (Ge1f), 64 (Li3), 72 (Mg7), 77 (Mo2), 88 (Pb3), 92 (S1f), 96 (Se1+3ff), 123 (Zn10f), 138, 141, 143 >> gout

K

Kayser-Fleischer corneal ring, 38 (Cu3f)

Keshan disease, vi, 98 (Se3f)

Kidney, 5 (Al2), 8 (As3), 12 (B1f), 17 (Be2), 19 (Bi2), 21 (Br2), 24 (Ca3f), 26 (Cd1ff), 38 (Cu3+5), 48 (Ge1f), 50 (Hg1ff), 60 (K1f), 63 (Li2ff), 66 (Mg1ff), 75 (Mn3), 80 (Na1),

83 (Ni2), 84 (P1f), 86 (Pb1f), 95 (Sb2), 97 (Se2ff), 103 (Si2f), 109 (Tl2), 123 (Zn10ff)

L

Laboratory, 5 (Al2), 35 (Cr2), 40 (Cu5), 64 (Li3), 68 (Mg3), 83 (Ni2), 8 5(Pb2), 113 (V2), 116 (Zn3+11), 128ff >> assessment and therapeutic application

Laxatives, 60 (K1), 66 (Mg1)

Lead, viii-x, 24 (Ca3), 27 (Cd2f), 43 (F2), 48 (Ge1f), 53 (Hg4f), 86 (Pb1ff), 107 (Sr2), 110 (Tl3), 114 (Zn1f+11), 129ff, 145, 152

Lithium, xii, 58 (I3), 62 (Li1ff), 110 (Tl3), 113 (V2), 129

Liver, 7 (As2f), 11 (Au2), 12 (B1f), 16 (Be1f), 27 (Cd2+4), 33 (Co2), 38 (Cu3ff), 47 (Fe3), 52 (Hg3), 72 (Mg7), 83 (Ni2), 92 (S1f), 96 (Se1f+4ff), 103 (Si2), 115 (Zn2+9ff), 132, 153

Lungs, 5 (Al2), 8 (As3), 12 (B1f), 15 (Ba2), 16 (Be1f), 20 (Br1f), 27 (Cd2ff), 33 (Co2), 35 (Cr2), 83 (Ni2), 91 (Pt2), 97 (Se2), 102 (Si1f), 105 (Sn2) 124 (Zn11ff), 153 >> acid/base regulation, silicosis

M

Magnesium, xiif, xvi, 4 (Al1f), 15 (Ba2), 24 (Ca3f), 40 (Cu5), 61 (K2), 63 (Li2), 66 (Mg1-7), 85 (P2), 86 (Pb1), 106 (Sr1f), 125 (Zn12), 128f, 134, 136, 141f

Manganese, xii, xvi, 45 (Fe1f), 73 (Mn1ff), 90 (Pt1), 114 (Zn1+6), 129, 135, 137, 141, 152

Mees' bands, 7-8 (As2f)

Memory, 3 (Ag2), 21 (Br2), 50 (Hg1), 52 (Hg3), 54 (Hg5), 119 (Zn6); compare ADHD, concentration, and IQ

Men/fertility, 47 (Fe3), 76 (Mo1ff), 88 (Pb3), 115 (Zn2ff)

Menkes' syndrome, 40 (Cu5)

Mercury, xiif, 3 (Ag2), 28 (Cd3), 43 (F2), 48 (Ge1f), 50 (Hg1ff), 96 (Se1+6), 104 (Sn1), 110 (Tl3), 124 (Zn11), 129ff

Metallothionein, 39 (Cu4), 55 (Hg6), 124 (Zn11), 126, 151

Migraine, 24 (Ca3), 39 (Cu4), 50 (Hg1+5), 62 (Li1+3), 66 (Mg1+3f) >> headaches

"Minamata disease", 52 (Hg3)

sensitivities, 54 (Hg5), 120 (Zn7)
thyroid function, 43 (F2), 56 (I1)
weight, 45 (Fe1), 119 (Zn6)
Prostaglandin metabolism, 64 (Li3), 70 (Mg5), 100 (Se5), 116 (Zn3+11)
Prostate, 117 (Zn4)
Protein, >> amino acids and enzymes
deficiency/loss, 28 (Cd3), 71 (Mg6), 73 (Mn1), 84 (P1), 93 (S2), 125 (Zn12)
intake (food sources), x, 73 (Mn1), 92 (S1f), 125 (Zn12)
metabolism, 73 (Mn1f), 115 (Zn2+6+11f), 150f
retinol binding, 122 (Zn9)
structural, 75 (Mn3), 93 (S2), 103 (Si2), 150
transport, 36 (Cu1+3f), 122 (Zn9)
transcription, 124 (Zn11)
zinc-dependant, 118 (Zn5f+9ff), 150f
zinc-finger protein, 124 (Zn11), 152
Psoriasis, 10 (Au1), 64 (Li3), 116 (Zn3+8+11)
Psychosis, 19 (Bi2), 21 (Br2), 39 (Cu4), 52 (Hg3), 65 (Li4), 68 (Mg3), 88 (Pb3), 109 (Tl2f), 122 (Zn9ff)

R

Radiation, xiii, 17 (Be2), 24 (Ca3), 27 (Cd2), 32 (Co1f), 59 (I4), 64 (Li3), 96 (Se1+5), 106 (Sr1f), 110 (Tl3), 114 (Zn1), 135, 153f
>> cancer (radiation therapy)
Recycling waste, 29 (Cd4), 110 (Tl3)
Reperfusion injury, 75 (Mn3), 101 (Se6)
>> strokes
Reproductive glands, 59 (I4), 115 (Zn2+10), 153
Retinol binding protein, 122 (Zn9)
Rust protectant, 27 (Cd2), 86 (Pb1)

S

Salt, xv, 14 (Ba1), 34 (Cr1f), 40 (Cu5), 58 (I3), 63 (Li2+4), 80 (Na1f), 91 (Pt2), 97 (Se2), 109 (Tl2), 119 (Zn6), 138
Selenium, vf, xiiff, 6 (As1), 29 (Cd4), 52 (Hg3ff), 59 (I4), 86 (Pb1), 90 (Pt1), 96 (Se1ff), 129, 131, 135ff, 141, 147
Selenosis, 96 (Se1f)

Sensory
hearing/deafness, 52 (Hg3), 116 (Zn3+10)
sensory-motor, 8 (As3), 33 (Co2), 52 (Hg3)
smell, 26 (Cd1+3), 93 (S2), 114 (Zn1+3+9)
taste, xiv, 28 (Cd3), 52 (Hg3), 93 (S2), 114 (Zn1+3+9f)
vision, 52 (Hg3+5), 70 (Mg5), 86 (Pb1), 116 (Zn3)
Sex hormones, 115 (Zn2+10), 151
>> estrogen
Sexual activity, 100 (Se5), 123 (Zn10)
Ships, 105 (Sn2)
Silicon, ix, xii, 102 (Si1f)
Silicosis, 5 (Al2), 35 (Cr2), 102 (Si1f)
Silver, (Ag1f), 11 (Au2), 21 (Br2), 53 (Hg4), 136, 147
Skin
acne, 20 (Br1f), 58 (I3), 121 (Zn8)
acrodermatitis enteropathica, 116 (Zn3+7+10)
diabetes, 121 (Zn8)
disorders, 114 (Zn1f)
elasticity, 13 (B2), 36 (Cu1f), 102 (Si1f), 121 (Zn8)
hyperkeratosis/parakeratosis, 8 (As3), 95 (Sb2), 115 (Zn2)
pallor/paleness, 8 (As3), 45 (Fe1), 86 (Pb1+3)
pigmentation, 3 (Ag2), 6 (As1+3), 11 (Au2), 18 (Bi1f), 40 (Cu5), 47 (Fe3), 94 (Sb1f)
rash, 8 (As3), 20 (Br1f), 83 (Ni2)
ulcers, 8 (As3), 35 (Cr2)
Sleep disorders/disturbances, 21 (Br2), 22 (Ca1), 57 (I2), 69 (Mg4), 86 (Pb1+3)
Smog, 7 (As2), 76 (Mo1f), 93 (S2)
Socioeconomic status, 109 (Tl2), 115 (Zn2+5)
Sodium, xii, xv, 21 (Br2), 30 (Cl1f), 61 (K2), 63 (Li2f), 80 (Na1f), 125 (Zn12), 130
Soil, v, vi, ix-xi, 13 (B2), 29 (Cd4), 33 (Co2), 44 (F3), 51 (Hg2), 57 (I2f), 77 (Mo2f), 97 (Se2f+5), 109 (Tl2), 117 (Zn4), 134, 140
fertilization, x, 12 (B1), 27 (Cd2+4),

ABOUT THE AUTHORS

Dr. med. Klaus-Georg Wenzel (born 1950) worked in the US during his medical education and passed the 1974 Educational Council for Foreign Medical Graduates (ECFMG) exam. He is a member of the International Society for Orthomolecular Medicine (ISOM), the German Anti-aging Society (GSAAM), and other societies. He also lectures in Europe and North America. Like his father (deceased), he specializes in neurology and psychiatry and has a private practice in Limburg, a town 60 miles north of Frankfurt. His additional fields of study include neurophysiology (including EEG-brain-mapping) and neuroorthopedics. Patients will often come to a specialist for help after having undergone other conventional medical treatments with little or no success. After several years in the medical profession, Dr. Wenzel learned from his patients the importance of using supplementary treatments, especially mineral and vitamin adjuncts. During his education as a physician in a hospital setting, he would see patients for a brief time and then lose contact with them, whether their conditions improved or not. In private practice he treated some patients for years and this long-term relationship instilled in him a moral obligation to look for other therapies not yet considered – or else why are you called a specialist? Medical practitioners should be able to investigate the cause of disease by considering the role of trace minerals in the assessment and treatment of patients. In recent years there has been an additional focus on biochemical and orthomolecular aspects of aging and neurodegenerative diseases including strokes and Parkinson's disease.

Dr. Raymond J Pataracchia, B.Sc., N.D. met Dr.Wenzel at an International Society for Orthomolecular Medicine (ISOM) conference and then visited him in Germany as a part of his medical internship. He has a 4 year honors degree in Neuroscience and four years of medical education from the Canadian College of Naturopathic Medicine, Toronto, Ontario. He is board (BDDT-N) certified in Ontario and has been in private practice in Toronto since 2002. His clinical focus is lab-based nutrition for psychiatric illness, cancer, and other conditions. His nutritional approach is described at www.nmrc.ca.

Resources for Patients and Healthcare Providers*

American Academy of Environmental Medicine, www.aaem.org Tel 316-684-5500

Canadian College of Naturopathic Medicine, 1255 Sheppard Avenue East, Toronto, Ontario, M2K 1E2, Tel. 416-498-1255, www.ccnm.edu

Institute of Holistic Nutrition, 18 Wyndford Drive, Unit 514, North York, Ontario, M3C 2S2, Tel. 416-386-0940

International Society for Orthomolecular Medicine, 16 Florence Ave., Toronto, Ontario, Canada, M2N 1E9 Tel: 416-733-2117 centre@orthomolecular.org

Alternative Therapies in Health and Medicine, alternative. therapies@innerdoorway.com

American Journal of Clinical Nutrition, www.ajcn.org

Integrative Medicine: A Clinician's Journal, www.imjournal.com

Journal of Nutritional & Environmental Medicine (UK), also available online

Journal of Orthomolecular Medicine, www.orthomed.org

Townsend Letter for Doctors And Patients, Tel 360-385-6021, tldp@olympus. net, www.tldp.com

MEDLINE (PubMed) provides intern access to all the world's medical literature; specific searches can be made easily.

www.garynull.com provides, for free, the complete data base up to 2004 of all medical literature on all minerals, vitamins, and essential nutrients; a cross-referenced data base available in 2006.

Laboratories offering hair and metabolic analyses for mineral and nutrient deficiencies

Anamol Laboratories, 83 Citation Drive, Unit # 9, Concord, Ontario, Canada, L4K 2Z6. Tel: 905-660-1225/ 1-888-254-4840, anamol@bellnet.ca, www.anamol.com

Doctor's Data, Chicago, Ill., 1-800-323-2784, inquiries@doctorsdata.com

Great Smokies Diagnostic Laboratory, USA 1-800-522-4762, www.gsdl.com, cs@gsdl.com

International Center Metabolic Testing, Ottawa, 1-888-591-4124

London Health Sciences Centre, Trace Elements Laboratory, 339 Windermere Rd, London, ON, N6A 5A5, Tel: 519-685-8500 (x35788)

Suppliers of plant-derived colloidal mineral supplements:

American Longevity www.americanlongevity.net US customers call 1-800-982-3193

Canadian branch of above coach@lifegetsbetter.info Canadian customers call 1-866-727-2191 Seroyal International Inc. Toronto, ON, 1-800-263-5861

Thorne Research, Inc., 1-800-228-1966

Signature Supplements Inc., 201 Brownlow Ave. unit 51, Dartmouth, NS, B3B 1W2 Tel. 902-435-7329 www.signaturesupplements.ca

* This list was compiled by Kos Publishing Inc as a service to readers of Kos books all of which contain resource information.

Books of Interest

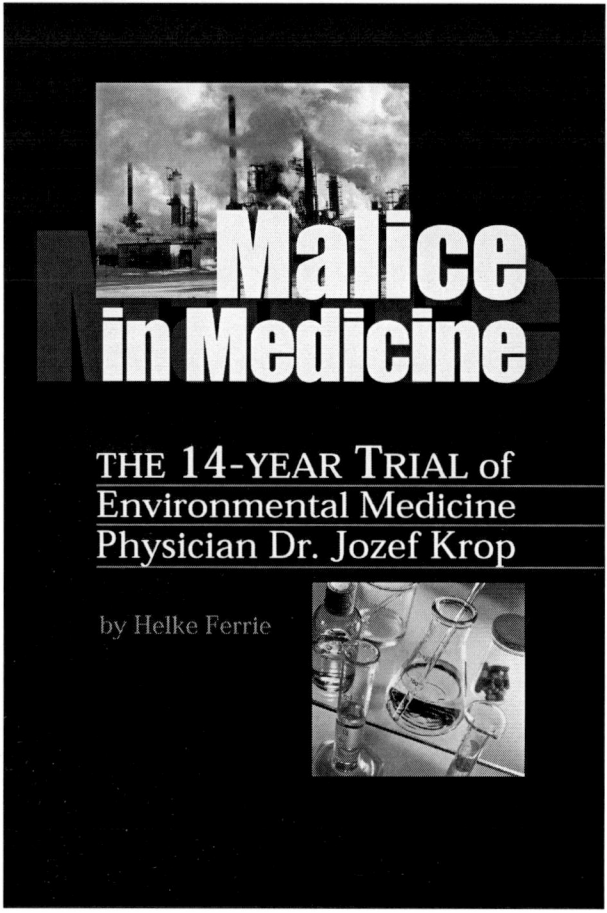

Malice in Medicine

THE 14-YEAR TRIAL of
Environmental Medicine
Physician Dr. Jozef Krop

by Helke Ferrie

From 1988 to 2002 Dr. Jozef Krop fought for the legal right to practice state-of-the-art environmental medicine. Without patient complaint, the prosecuting College of Physicians and Surgeons of Ontario (mandated to control doctors' licenses) maintained that environmentally induced illness is at best a psychiatric disorder and ignored international medical consensus on Multiple Chemical Sensitivity, Sick Building Syndrome and related medical conditions. Dr. Krop's battle was supported by a stellar international panel of medical experts and by thousands of patients made ill by industrial chemicals and pesticides; legal costs exceeded 1 million dollars, all paid by public donations. This book tells the dramatic story of a physician's successful challenge of corruption in the medical regulatory system.

6" × 9" | 400 pages | PB | $25.00
November 2005

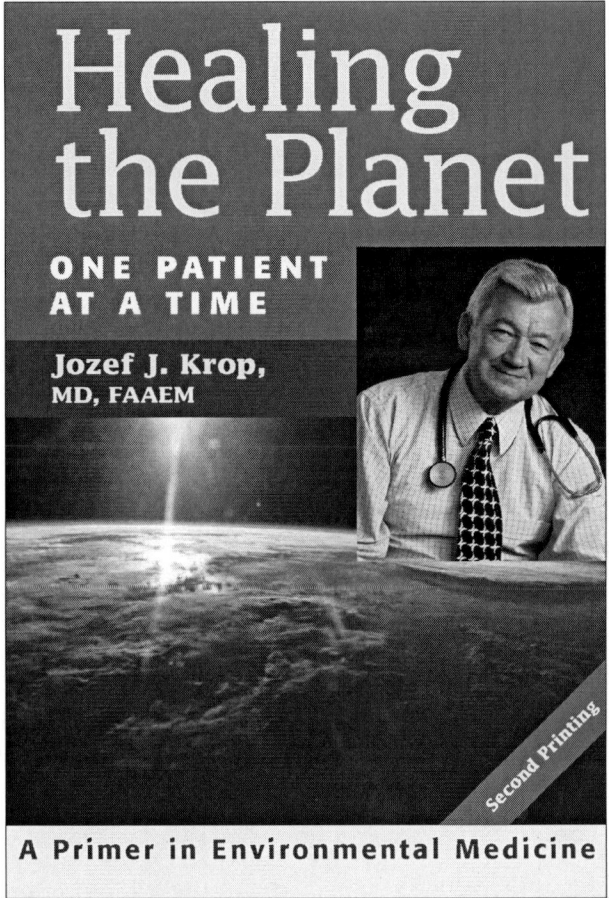

Healing the Planet

ONE PATIENT AT A TIME

Jozef J. Krop, MD, FAAEM

Second Printing

A Primer in Environmental Medicine

The general reader learns from his book to:
- identify health hazards in the home and work-place environments and what to do about them
- find help through a comprehensive resource section covering everything from pesticides to food allergies, electromagnetic fields, holistic dentistry, safe building materials, how to become a practitioner in environmental medicine and much more
- recognize warning signs that indicate probable environmental illness and how to find medically reliable help

Readers who are health professionals may use this book
- to find the references from the mainstream medical literature covering the field of environmental toxins and the treatment of environmental illness
- basic treatment and detoxification protocols for patients with environmental illness

ISBN 0-9731945-0-2
6" × 9" | 368 pages | PB | $25.00 | 2003

Books of Interest

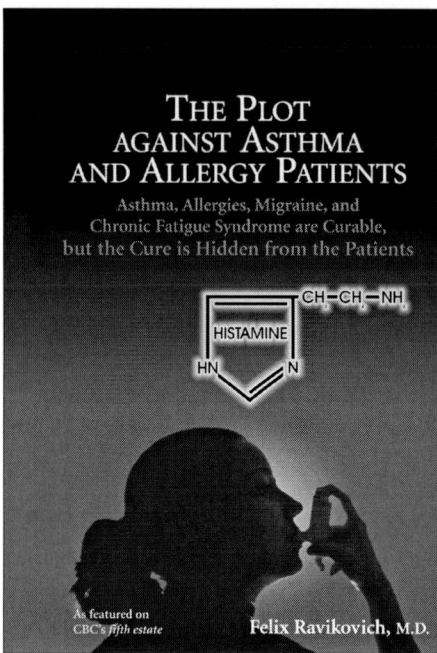

THE PLOT
AGAINST ASTHMA
AND ALLERGY PATIENTS

Asthma, Allergies, Migraine, and
Chronic Fatigue Syndrome are Curable,
but the Cure is Hidden from the Patients

HISTAMINE

As featured on
CBC's *fifth estate*   Felix Ravikovich, M.D.

DR. FELIX RAVIKOVICH obtained his medical degree and specialized in Internal Medicine in the former Soviet Union. Since 1985, he has practiced in Toronto specializing in allergy and asthma. His presentations at international conferences on the effective treatment with h i stamine were published in leading medical journals. This is his first book for the general public and medical colleagues.

Dr. Ravikovich describes his clinical experience with histamine—a synthetic version of the body's substance that stimulates the body to heal itself. His histamine therapy freed hundreds of asthma, allergy and migraine sufferers from drugs that have disastrous effects on the patients' health and the course of the diseases for which these drugs are prescribed.

Unlike other books that concentrate on triggers, this book spells out the primary cellular and genetic defects in patients with allergies, asthma and related diseases and shows how to repair these defects. The author substantiates this through the theoretical works of the world's leading scientists.

Dr. Ravikovich undertook an extensive detective search of literature in molecular biology, immuno-pharmacology, genetics, and clinical medicine that led him to unprecedented revelations. The scientific foundation for the treatment that could save millions from suffering and dying has been concealed by the medical elite to enable the pharmaceutical industry to develop only those drugs that do not cure and ensure indefinite patient dependence.

Dr. Ravikovich tells the story of his own battle with the medical regulatory authorities which work actively to suppress good, scientifically grounded medicine and protect—not patients—but corporate interests.

ISBN 0-9731945-1-0 | 2003
6" × 9" | 432 pages | PB | $25.00

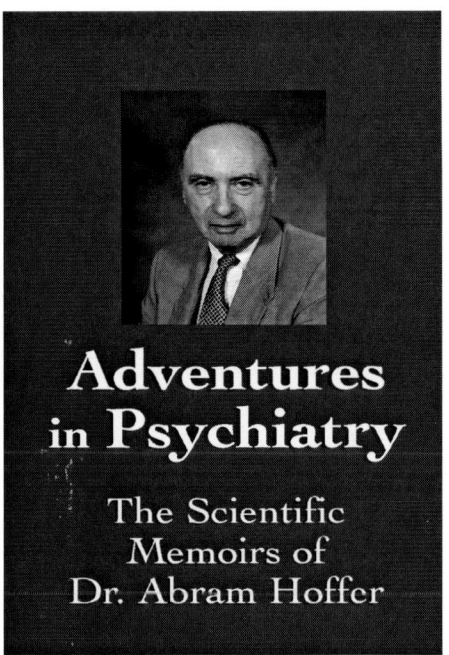

Adventures in Psychiatry

The Scientific Memoirs of Dr. Abram Hoffer

This book is a feast for the mind and the spirit: the autobiography of one of the great doctors of the 20th century, Dr. Abram Hoffer. For those of us who have learned, through painful personal experience that drugs, surgery, and most of high-tech medicine offer only very temporary benefits, but rarely if ever a cure, this book tells the wonderful story of the rebirth of nutritional medicine. Based on the science of biochemistry, now known as orthomolecular medicine.

Here we follow the journey of its founder: from his Saskatchewan farm childhood, subsequent training in bio-chemistry and agricultural science, his early insights into the central importance to human and animal health of soil and plant food quality, to his specialization in psychiatry, professorship at the University of Saskatchewan, and his daily work with patients. We learn of his disillusionment with traditional methods of treating the mentally ill and we share his excitement of discovery as we follow his dramatic case histories, which unfold like detective-stories, as he uncovers the connection between deficiencies in specific vitamins, minerals and essential fatty acids and mental illness. Once teamed up with the great Linus Pauling, we re-live their research odysseys that led to modern orthomolecular medicine, transforming psychiatry, the treatment of cancer and chronic disease, and offering patients recovery, not merely death-watch maintenance therapies. In addition to Dr. Hoffer's many fruitful years working with Pauling, we also meet many colleagues who helped design the rigorous research programs for orthomolecular medicine.

ISBN 0-9731945-X-X

6" x 9" | PB | $30.00

Books of Interest

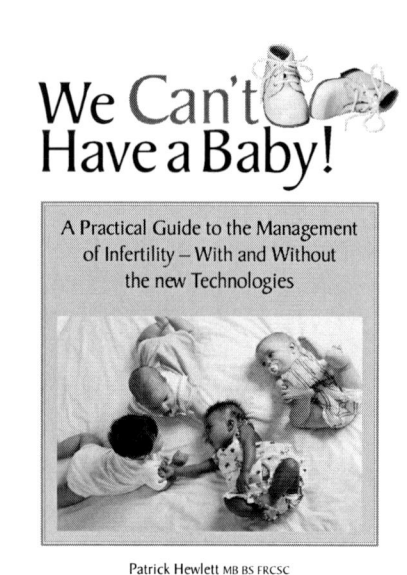

We Can't Have a Baby!

A Practical Guide to the Management of Infertility – With and Without the new Technologies

Patrick Hewlett MB BS FRCSC

This book is intended to help those couples who find themselves confronted with their inability to have a baby.

Infertility is usually defined as "inability to conceive after twelve months of intercourse without contraception" but common sense is needed. If there is an obvious problem, for example related to a previous attack of pelvic infection and damage of the Fallopian tubes, then investigation and management should not be delayed. If the wife is in her late thirties or early forties, assessment should be done without waiting one year. In the absence of other factors, six months without contraception is long enough to wait before getting a professional opinion from your family doctor.

This book will guide you through the many problems you will encounter and will provide you with information to help you make informed decisions about the best management in your own personal situation. Some sections provide precise options for management and others provide more general information depending on the relevance of the information for the couple.

Probably the most important aspect of helping with the problem of infertility is to ensure that enough time and expertise are used to make rational decisions about management. It makes no sense to access the latest and most complicated technology just because you are seen in a high-technology unit and want the "latest treatment." Your management depends on sensible decisions being made with the help of competent professionals. Very simple changes may be all that is needed even in some couples with long-standing infertility. I have seen couples who have even been through in-vitro fertilization cycles when subsequent successful pregnancy followed simple advice about life-style changes or simple medical management of readily identifiable abnormalities.

ISBN 0-9731945-4-5 | 2005
6" × 9" | PB | $25.00

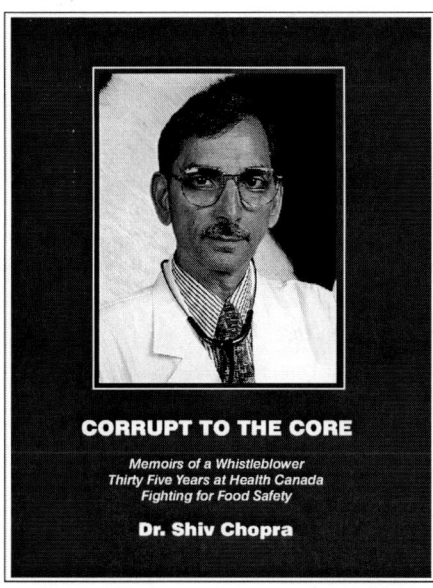

CORRUPT TO THE CORE

Memoirs of a Whistleblower
Thirty Five Years at Health Canada
Fighting for Food Safety

Dr. Shiv Chopra

Dr. Shiv Chopra' s name has become synonymous with food safety. Dr. Chopra and some of his fellow scientists waged many battles over many years against a succession of Canadian federal ministries of health—theft employer.

With full support of The Professional Institute of the Public Service of Canada—a 50,000 member union of scientific and professional public service employees, Dr. Chopra and his colleagues refused to approve various harmful drugs to be used in meat and milk production. Despite the political pressures to do otherwise, and holding fast to sound science, they did better than the gambles that a series of prime ministers and health ministers played with public safety.

Time and again the federal courts supported Dr. Chopra and his fellow scientists and ruled against government attempts to shut them up. Also, time and again the government over-ruled these scientists to feed corporate greed and allowed dangerous drugs to enter food production. Yet, today, the dangers of these drugs are internationally recognized and many countries have forbidden their use for such purposes. In 1999, Bovine Growth Hormone was barred in Canada and in the European Union, which was due essentially to Dr. Chopra's negative findings on this drug going back to 1988. Since 2000, the United States government has been trying unsuccessfully to withdraw market approval for a very seriously hazardous antibiotic, Baytril for which regulatory compliance in Canada was rejected by Dr. Chopra in 1995.

Here is the full account of how government corruption endangers the public food supply and how Dr. Chopra and his colleagues fearlessly continue to "to speak truth to power." Here is also the story of how the elected representatives in both Canada and USA are more interested in protecting industrial profits and trade, instead of the public's health. The stories told here for the first time include products like Revalor-H, Baytril, Bovine Growth Hormone, Silicon Breast Implants, and slaughterhouse waste to cause the biggest ruin of health safety—Bovine Spongiform Encephalopathy (BSE) or "mad-cow disease."

Everybody who eats should read this book.

ISBN 0-9731945-7-X | 2005 | November | 6" × 9" | PB | $30.00

$40 w/CD which contains media interviews, government documents, federal court decisions, scientific bibliographies and more.

Books of Interest

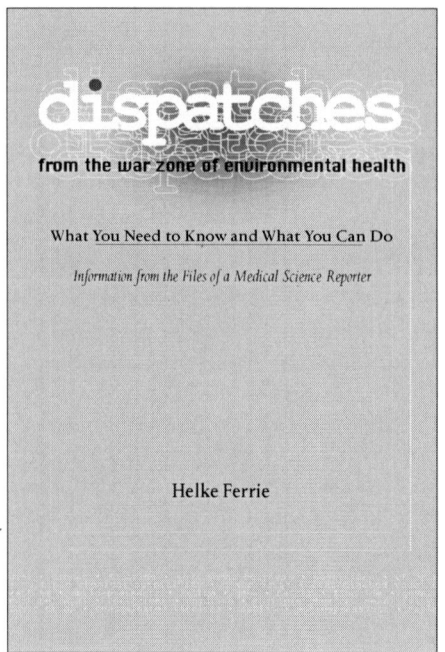

The weapons of mass destruction have been found, at least in medicine, and only we—the people, the consumers, the patients—can stop their proliferation by rouge corporations and their buddies in government. We have known about them for a long time actually, but their origins have been attributed to different sources over time. In antiquity, malevolent deities were thought responsible for the plagues that wiped out city-states and later caused economic disaster for the Roman Empire. In the Middle Ages, God was believed to be angry with sinful humanity and therefore visited epidemics on them, as he was believed to have done in the biblical stories about the Egypt at the time of Moses. In the mid-19th century, the poor of the vast slums associated with Europe's great cities were blamed for spreading mysterious diseases whose bacterial and viral causes were not yet understood by science.

Today, we know that the weapons of mass destruction are human-made chemicals, causing our current plague of chronic and degenerative diseases, and they are found in those substances intended to kill bugs, slugs, dandelions as well as in most of the drugs manufactured to fight cancer, impotence, heart disease, a rthritis and other illnesses. These chemicals are the basis of an amoral economic system that sells toxic chemicals in all their forms with the promise of perfect lawns, p e rfect agricultural produce, perfectly hygienic kitchens, perfect white laundry, and perfect magic-bullet drugs. In fact, they harm us and are guaranteed to harm coming generations as well. Marketing techniques ensure that the whole truth is as carefully disguised as possible. That truth being, that our chemically saturated food, air, water, and soil are the sources of all our diseases—either directly, or by compromising our immune responses, or by giving pathogens the evolutionary advantage.

ISBN 0-9731945-3-7 | PB
336 pages | $25.00 CDN

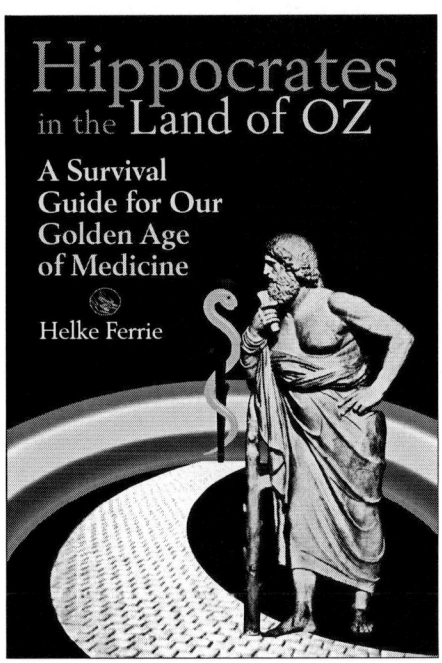
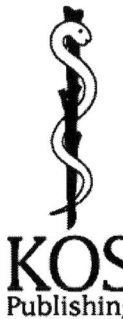

KOS
Publishing

KOS Publishing Inc. is named after the Greek island where the father of modern medicine, Hippocrates, was born 2,500 years ago. Our books are dedicated to the hope that current developments in medicine will constitute a rebirth, in modern contexts, of ancient insights into the centrality of environment and nutrition. Our books hope to educate and empower readers in the politics of medicine and provide helpful information on non-toxic medicine based on basic science and clinical proof.

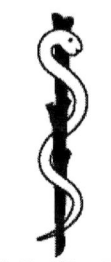

Order form

KOS can be contacted at the address given below to obtain more information or to place an order for any of our publications.

KOS PUBLISHING INC.
1997 Beechgrove Road,
Alton, Ontario Canada L0N 1A0
Tel: (519) 927-1049
Fax: (519) 927-9542
Email: helke@inetsonic.com • info@kospublishing.com

Name: _____   Date: _____

Address: _____   Payment: ◯ Cheque ◯ Visa

City: _____   ◯ Master Card

Prov./State: _____   Name on Card: _____

Postal/Zip Code: _____   Card #: _____

Telephone: _____   Expiry Date: _____

Email: _____   Signature: _____

ISBN	TITLE	QTY.	PRICE	TOTAL
0-9731945-0-2	Healing the Planet		$25.00	
0-9731945-1-0	The Plot Against Asthma and Allergy Patients		$25.00	
0-9731945-2-9	Hippocrates in the Land of Oz		$25.00	
0-9731945-3-7	Dispatches From the War Zone of En v i ronmental Health		$25.00	
0-9731945-4-5	We Can't Have a Baby!		$25.00	
0-9731945-X-X	Adventures in Psychiatry		$30.00	
0-9731945-5-3	The Gift of the Earth		$25.00	
0-9731945-7-X	Corrupt to the Core		$30.00	
0-9731945-7-X	Corrupt to the Core with CD		$40.00	

Shipping Charges: 1 title $6.00, for each additional title add $3 plus GST. Bulk orders of 10 copies or more of any *one title* receive a 50% discount on books only, regular shipping and taxes apply.

SUB-TOTAL	
TAXES	
TOTAL	